HOW TO BE
A GOD-PLEASING
PATIENT

HOW TO BE A GOD-PLEASING PATIENT

A BIBLICAL APPROACH TO RECEIVING MEDICAL CARE

DR. JIM HALLA

Ambassador International
GREENVILLE, SOUTH CAROLINA & BELFAST, NORTHERN IRELAND

www.ambassador-international.com

How to Be a God-Pleasing Patient

A Biblical Approach to Receiving Medical Care

ISBN: 978-1-62020-905-9

eISBN: 978-1-62020-918-9

Cover Design and Page Layout by Hannah Nichols

Ebook Conversion by Anna Riebe Raats

AMBASSADOR INTERNATIONAL

411 University Ridge Suite B14

Greenville, SC 29609, USA

www.ambassador-international.com

AMBASSADOR BOOKS

The Mount

2 Woodstock Link

Belfast, BT6 8DD, Northern Ireland, UK

www.ambassador-international.com

The colophon is a trademark of Ambassador

Contents

Preface

DAILY LIVING CAN BE UNPLEASANT—ESPECIALLY when our bodies are not working like we want. Being a patient is not always easy and most of my patients agree. Several factors influence being a patient. There is the medical condition itself with its unpleasantness, misery, and uncertainty. There is the effort and time involved in receiving medical care. There are financial aspects as part of the burden of illness. You could probably think of many more.

In response to failing bodies, people seek various kinds of help from many sources. These include doctors, the Internet, self-help books, mother or some other family member. Nevertheless, it seems "American" to visit the doctor. Americans are encouraged to go to the doctor by any number of groups that stress both prevention and treatment.

Visiting the doctor usually begins at birth and it is often the last thing one does. It is reported that four out of five Americans say that they "feel sick" in any given month, and one in five will visit a doctor's office. It is estimated that there are 400 million visits to a doctor per year and another 425 million visits to providers of alternative care [1](these providers *are not*

1.Reisser, PC; Mabe, D; Velarde, P: *Examining Alternative Medicine: An Inside Look at the Benefits and Risks;* InterVarsity Press, Downers Grove, Illinois, 2001, p. 17.

necessarily physicians). It is safe to say that most Americans will be a patient sometime during their lifetime.

People go to the doctor for a variety of reasons. Many want to stay healthy and seek information on preventive measures such as lifestyle changes, nutrition, exercise and activity, and various medications. Others want treatment for various ailments. And still others want to make sure there is nothing wrong with their bodies. Sadly, there are only a handful of patients who will visit the doctor in order to be a good steward of the body that God has entrusted to them. These few desire to honor God by taking care of their bodies His way for His glory. As a result, they may also reap the benefit of improved health in this present life.

The real issue for many believers is this: how we do live this life with a myriad of problems including physical ones. Patients often tell me that they understand that complaining about health problems is a complaint against God. They also tell me that they are looking forward to heaven and their glorified bodies. However, many have little hope for this life unless problems, any and all, cease. They fail to connect the hope and anticipation of a glorified body with living as a God-pleaser using their problems to become more Christlike. Complaints against God are sinful, dishonor God, and are not conducive to improved health. Becoming more like Christ does not often motivate them to look forward and upward. It was in that way, that Jesus left heaven, took on human flesh, marched to the cross, and remained there. He lived well so He would die well. Believers imitate Christ when they maintain a Godward focus and an eternal perspective. In that way they are of earthly good and experience the joy of being God's child, even if they have failing bodies. Many times, believers fail to enjoy what they are in Christ indwelt by the Holy Spirit. Consequently, they are burdened and disenchanted; physical problems may worsen, and the Holy Spirit is grieved.

The hope of a resurrected, glorified body is a motivating factor in being God's kind of patient (1 Corinthians 15:42-49). Earlier in the same chapter Paul wrote that if only for this life we hope in Christ, we are to be pitied (v.19). This hope of a glorified body and eternal living is often not considered as a blessing now—in the believer's present life. Sometimes believers view death and salvation as a fire escape out of hell or from hell on earth. However, the believer's hope is not primarily a glorified body, appealing as that is. We still have a life to live until Jesus returns. Rather, the believer's true hope is an everlasting one. It is being in the presence of the Triune God. God desires and deserves to have His people to be in His presence, but they must be clothed suitably for the occasion. Before they receive their glorified bodies—they must have the proper wedding garments—Christ's righteousness—at which time their bodies will be glorified (Matthew 22:1-14; Romans 3:22; 2 Corinthians 5:21; Philippians 1:9; 3:9). It seems that the believer's glorified body is more for God than it is for the believer! In heaven, the believer reaps the joy of being in God's presence, but the believer must be dressed for the occasion!

In this life, the believer still with his unglorified body looks ahead to being in God's glorious presence. This forward, vertical, and eternal perspective is an essential element of being a believer and is the result of the daily presence of God via the

Holy Spirit and the believer's union with Christ. The foretaste of heaven and future glory as described above enables believers to view themselves and their earthly bodies from a completely different perspective and live on this earth accordingly. Resurrection and eternal life begins at salvation and enables and encourages believers to practice biblical stewardship as godly theologians (Romans 6:9-10; 1 John 3:1-3). The theology of the patient as well as the physician matters. Living well as a godly patient and as a godly physician is the one way to die well.

Christian friend, if you are not in that last category, let me raise a matter that you may not have considered—*your* relationship with Christ. That relationship should impact every aspect of your life and should influence your reasons for visiting a doctor and how you function as a patient. The reality of your relationship with Christ sets you apart from the unbelieving patient in the next examining room.

Reader, if you are not a Christian, then this book can be a blessing to you as well. The application of biblical truth always simplifies life. However, unless the Holy Spirit has taken up residence in your heart, you don't have the proper receiving set to hear and properly respond to God's truth about you, Himself, your body, and living in God's world. I encourage you to keep reading and perhaps God will use the book as a vehicle for you to come to Him. That is one of my prayers!

Introduction

THE TRUTH OF ONE'S RELATIONSHIP with Christ affecting all of life applies to both the physician and patient alike. I have written a book that addresses how the doctor's relationship with Christ impacts their ability to be a doctor God's way.[2] While that book may be of interest to you, this book is addressed specifically to every patient who is a believer.

Too often the patient's relationship with Christ doesn't affect how they think about being a patient, their body, and how they respond to and utilize the doctor's advice. And it should! As we shall see, theology matters! Therefore, I want you to consider the truth that being a patient God's way is best for you and honors God. My two-fold goal in writing this book is:

1. To help you be God's kind of patient.

2. To help you minister to your doctor.

In order to accomplish this goal, we must develop a proper view and theology of being a patient. That may sound strange. Therefore, I unpack that concept in the book. As I do, you will discover what God says in the Bible about taking care of the body. Having done that, we will look at ways to apply those biblical principles in your own life as a patient.

---

2. I have written books addressing this question from the doctor's side entitled, *True Competence in Medicine: Practicing Biblically-Based Medicine in a Fallen World* and *Being Christian in Your Medical Practice*. You may want to read them and/or give them to your doctor.

Briefly stated, being a patient God's way is taking care of yourself His way. Man is not simply a body. He is a whole person—inner (the non-material aspect of man) and outer man (the material, physical aspect of man). Man is a unit. The outer man is influenced by what is in the inner man and vice versa. Since our bodies are a gift from God taking care of it is a privilege and blessing as well as a duty. Therefore, it should be for His honor and glory. Good stewardship of our body should be motivated by the desire to thankfully please Him. Staying healthy, relief, and "getting cured" are not to be our main goal; these are only potential by-products of being a patient God's way.

Being a patient God's way in part means using biblical principles in order to think, desire, and act correctly in caring for the whole person—body and soul. As a result, we will go to the doctor with the correct motivation and willingness to hear about the problem and a proposed solution. After receiving the doctor's conclusions, we will seek to understand what has been said and then carry out a solution according to biblical principles. Throughout the book, I will present examples of what being a patient God's way looks like.

This definition flows from the often neglected but foundational facts that all of life is theological and everyone is a theologian. Since every person has beliefs about God and is in a proper or improper relationship with Him, he is a theologian and he practices theology. These two truths convey the reality that life is lived vertically—in relationship to God as a believer or apart from God as an unbeliever. Therefore, the believer's relationship with Christ must influence all of life including being a patient.

A good theologian seeks God's kingdom first (Matthew 6:33). They do that by faithfully honoring God whether the body is failing or not. Functioning as a good theologian may include going to the physician but always as a good steward. We must remember that healing, relief, and or good health may or may not be the result of good stewardship. Believers know that the result of biblical stewardship is not our prerogative—it is God's. However, obedient believers will use what they don't like to become more like Christ. How can that be true? The believer who desires to be a patient God's way has realized one lesson of the cross: Jesus used what is considered repulsive and bad for good—the redemption of His people (1 Corinthians 1:18-31). Jesus redeemed His people through His perfect life and His prefect but brutal death. The believer-patient, called to imitate his Lord, will also use what the doesn't like for good which is always defined according to Scripture. The good is growth in Christlikeness as the believer uses his failing body to become more like Christ.

In the process of going to the physician as a good steward, the believer may receive unwanted or even potentially devastating information. During this situation, the Christian is faced with unpleasantness and uncertainty. Fortified with the truth that God is in control and works for both His glory and the believer's benefit, the believer will embrace the situation in God's strength rather than his own. He will develop increasing trust in and dependence on a marvelously good God. The cross and Christ's resurrection prove that fact. Like Christ, the believer does not simply cope, accept the situation, tolerate, or "suck it up." Rather the Christian knows that God's purpose for him is to glorify God which is done by pleasing Him by growing in Christlikeness. And since Christ was the ultimate God pleaser, the believer imitates Him especially when life is hard. More than anyone else, the Christian recognizes and acts upon God's truth that victory is becoming more like Christ rather than getting relief. Like Christ, the believer has an eternal perspective such that they endure to the end.

The believer is also aware that the kingdom of God is more than physical relief and pleasures such as eating and drinking. It is peace, joy, and righteousness (Romans 14:17). He is in God's kingdom as a result of a radical, supernatural transfer from Satan's family and kingdom into God's (Colossians 1:13-14). One purpose of this new membership is becoming more like Christ, Who purchased the believer and his failing body with His own broken, bloodied body. Therefore, the believer is not his own. His Savior is now his *Master* (1 Corinthians 6:19-20; 7:23). Therefore, taking care of one's body God's way for God's sake is what a good theologian-steward does. In that way, he honors the *Master*.

In the preceding paragraphs I have laid out basic and foundational truths for functioning as God's kind of patient. However, the believer, while a saint (one set apart for Christ by Christ through the Holy Spirit), is not perfected. We often view circumstances including failing bodies from the perspective of feelings and "I wants." When that happens, we have veered from biblical truth. The tunnel seems so long, the mountain so high, and the hole so deep. It is then, and even prior to this downward spiral, that we must counsel ourselves. We must call ourselves back to our God. God is the Comforter, yet He is more than that. He is the Creator, Controller, and Sustainer of His people. I will refer back to these truths and a proper use of them throughout the book.

However, if one's motive is merely to get relief he is functioning as a poor theologian-steward and thereby using God and displeasing Him. When relief doesn't come, there is the temptation to use God's providence as an excuse to show displeasure in a variety of ways. The temptation is great, but it must be avoided. A proper vertical, eternal, and upward focus is one of God's tools for the believer to use in order to please God even when believers don't think they can. One common response to God's providence—for instance a failing body or poor health—is grumbling and complaining and the excuses that believers use to justify this response (Philippians 2:14-17). At its core, the grumbler and complainer suggest that Christ has failed to do His job at the cross and that the Father has failed to treat the person better than He treated His Son. Either way, the believer-patient will find little comfort for this life or the life to come if he approaches being a patient as a poor theologian.

In contrast, good theologians know that satisfaction and contentment in this life only come from viewing and responding to things God's way for His glory. The theologian-steward applies one of the lessons of the cross by using what a person doesn't like for daily growth in Christlikeness. This approach to daily living is at the core of being God's kind of person and patient. Believer, please ask and answer the question: which kind of theologian are you? This book is designed to help you function as a godly patient-theologian.

Why Go to the Doctor

THERE ARE MANY REASONS FOR going to a doctor. How is a person to decide the proper reason for going? We must turn to the Bible. Your first reaction to this exhortation may be an incredulous: The Bible! Yes, the Bible. How do I arrive at that conclusion? Regarding the body, salvation does not completely remove the effects of the curse of sin in this life (Romans 5:12-14; 2 Corinthians 4:16-18). On earth before Christ's return, every person's body fails with resultant misery and death.[3] Everyone in varying degrees experiences the result of the curse of sin. These facts mean that you must consider your body and medical care from a different perspective than the culture does. You must turn to the Bible which is in your best interest and is absolutely necessary for you to learn how to honor God. The faithful application of God's truth does that. "Bad" bodies should not, and do not, remove the joy, privilege, and blessing of being a child of God and using physical conditions as a means to grow and change.

The Bible is inspired by the One Who created and designed man. God designed man as a whole person, body and soul. He beckons believers to read and understand His truth (Isaiah

---

3. See my article: "What do you do when your body fails you?" available at my website: jimhalla.com.

8:19-20). While the Bible is not a medical textbook, it does give Christians everything they need for eternal life and godly living here (2 Peter 1:3-4). Therefore, all the principles needed to be a God-honoring patient are contained within Scripture. Seeking God's answers from the Bible is non-negotiable. Answers found elsewhere may be *counterfeit wisdom.* Believers must go to the Bible because it is God's manual for life.

Having decided to go to the doctor, will you go as a wise and good theologian or a poor and foolish one? Unfortunately, too many Christians visit the physician with the same mindset as unbelievers. My hope in writing this book is to help all believers develop a God-honoring mindset as they seek health care. Consider the fact that the surrounding presence of God makes it impossible for anyone to be theologically and morally neutral (Psalm 139). To try to be neutral is attempting to remove God from a part of your life.

Taking care of the body is a theological-moral issue involving a standard and a goal. This means that going to the doctor is a theological-moral issue. For Christians, the two can never be separated. Examining the motivation for going to the doctor is important if a person is to function as God's kind of patient. So, too, is a person's expectation and definition of help. Patients seeking help typically have expectations and perceived ideas of what is wrong and the help they want. Some even have an agenda for getting help. Normally it is relief—"get me well." In those cases, the person desires to have the doctor function as a "body mechanic" with the goal of making "me feel better." At other times, a patient will go to the doctor out of desperation or even fear. Sometimes when times are difficult, the believer-patient may function as if they have lost the goal of pleasing

God. Functionally, they have rejected the truth that pleasing God doesn't guarantee relief.

In these scenarios the key is God's agenda rather than the person's or the doctor's. God's kind of stewardship can and must be practiced even if pain relief or cure doesn't result from visiting the doctor. God's grace is sufficient (1 Corinthians 10:13; 2 Corinthians 12:7-10). Getting relief, as I have said, is a by-product of being a good steward rather than the primary goal, hope, and expectation.

CHAPTER 1

The Goal of Going
to the Doctor

A PATIENT GENERALLY COMES TO the doctor with one of two goals: diagnosis and treatment or prevention and maintenance of health and physical function. The patient has thoughts, desires, and expectations about his problem, himself, and his doctor that affect how he will function as a patient. In fact, patients live out of an identity. They have labeled themselves in a certain way and it affects how they think and act. For instance, patients may consider themselves a cancer sufferer—or perhaps a cancer survivor. That identity will have important implications as he or she visits the doctor as well as throughout life.

Sometimes both the problem and the treatment solution will be clear. If the problem is acute such as tonsillitis or appendicitis, the treatment solution is generally antibiotics or surgery, respectively. These acute illnesses are usually curable. Once the patient is better or cured, he often forgets the problem existed. In these situations, it is easy for the patient to neglect or seemingly forget his relationship with Christ except perhaps, to thank God for healing. He functions as if his response to the condition was not significantly influenced by his relationship with Christ. He may think that unbelievers are healed so why not him.

At other times the problem may not be so simple. The diagnosis may be difficult, the treatment hard, or the condition long lasting. Chronic diseases come in many shapes and sizes, and the daily reality of their presence may be consuming. No matter the problem, the believer-patient may be so focused on relief, cure, maintaining health, or preventing "bad health" that going to the doctor, taking various remedies, and engaging in lifestyle changes becomes a way of life. The person may function as if cure is expected because "God is working through the doctor." God uses secondary causes including physicians and various treatments and often healing comes. But God also heals unbelievers and not every believer is healed. Pleasing God through good stewardship is to be the believer's goal. The results are God's prerogative and often an added blessing to and for good stewardship.

Consider the believer. All believers are to function as good theologians no matter the circumstances in which God has placed them. That is the key: God's control is good even when the circumstances and a person's feelings seem to scream otherwise. God is good all the time, and a person's circumstances do not change that truth. Moreover, God is powerful as well as good. Therefore, the believer, and only the believer, can function as a good theologian. His relationship with Christ should take center stage in helping him get victory in all of life including health problems. True victory is defined biblically as being controlled by biblical principles and not by his wants or the agony of his condition; it is using the condition to become more like Christ; and it is pleasing God rather than seeking relief. Victory God's way is the only way that brings great satisfaction and contentment in the face of tremendous unpleasantness.

CHAPTER 2
At the Doctor's Office

So, YOU HAVE GONE TO the doctor! Now what? Once at the doctor's office, what treatment might you receive? It depends on several variables including your condition, your desires and thoughts about the situation, and the physician's diagnosis and treatment plan. Since patients are seeking answers and relief, it is easy for both the patient and physician to focus on relief only. If the patient and the doctor believe that every symptom has a cause, the doctor will look for one. He begins by asking questions. The doctor will perform a physical examination, often obtain blood work, and do radiographic studies. The physician is hunting for a cause of the patient's problems in hopes of prescribing a visible, tangible treatment.

If no cause is found additional studies may be done depending on the type of problem and physician visited. If the problem is thought to be musculoskeletal or neurological, MRI and CAT scans may be ordered. Complaints of undiagnosed chest pain may result in a cardiac (heart) or gastrointestinal (gut) workup. If no cause is discovered, the patient's symptoms may be attributed to an "emotional" or "psychiatric" disturbance and treatment begun on that basis. Often the major goal in all these endeavors is to bring about relief from symptoms and bad feelings.

Reader, you may be wondering: is it bad, let alone wrong, to seek relief? Often, people ask me if it is wrong to want to feel better and to dislike feeling bad. The quick answer is not necessarily. But any good desire, if desired too much or pursued sinfully, is wrong, not necessarily the desire itself, but the effort to get it and the response to not getting it. Therefore, these types of questions must bring us back to the Bible and the cross. Christ saved sinners by living a perfectly righteous life and dying a perfect death. His body was brutally broken for the salvation of His people in order to honor His Father. But His work in life and death didn't guarantee a life without physical problems for anyone. Even the creation knows that the full redemption of the body awaits Jesus' return (Romans 8:19-22).

The Bible exhorts and encourages the believer to take care of his body God's way and for His glory with the purpose of pleasing Him (Romans 6:6; 1 Corinthians 6:19-20;7:23; 10:31; 2 Corinthians 5:9-15). When believers go to the doctor with that mindset and perspective, God is honored. Believers reap the benefit of knowing that he has returned to God his body, as part of a whole-person activity, which God has entrusted to him (1 Corinthians 6:19-20; 7:23).

Now, armed with God's perspective, we can answer the question: "Is it right to take care your body?" with certainty and Amen! God would have it no other way. The Bible also points out that biblical stewardship doesn't guarantee relief. The result of good stewardship is in the hands of God. We are to leave the results to the Lord. Christ wasn't guaranteed relief by the Father, so why should we expect to be treated differently than God treated His Son?

A bit more on the issue of relief. There are three general treatment approaches that you may be faced with when going to the doctor. One is what is called traditional medicine. This approach includes conventional treatment regimens including medications and surgery. Most physicians believe these to be proven and therefore acceptable. Another approach is the use of alternative medicine which includes natural foods and nutrients such as vitamins and supplements. As a rule, these products have received less scientific study and scrutiny. A third is the use of spirituality which may be added to your treatment regimen. Far too often the term spirituality has nothing to do with biblical truth. If your goal is solely or inordinately to live a healthy, normal life, you may be tempted to rely on sources exclusive of the Bible. You must avoid this temptation. One reason I am developing a theology of being a patient God's way is to help counter these temptations. Biblical truth is not opposed to scientific truth nor is it opposed to taking care of the body. In fact, practicing biblical truth is the best way for the believer to take care of his body (Proverbs 3:5-8).

Let us consider some thoughts about medications and relief. Since we live in a consumer-driven society, medications are ever before the public. Often drug treatments are first introduced by the media to the patient-consumer. This has the effect of stimulating patients to contact the physician's office with inquiries about specific drugs that are advertised as having the potential of curing or improving the person's symptoms or condition. While drug treatment may be an example of good stewardship of one's body, it may also serve simply to change feelings unrelated to any change in the body. When that happens, both the patient and physician may lose sight of the primary reason a believer should go to the doctor: to honor God by functioning as a good steward. Man is not his feelings, yet he is taught that he is. One of culture's primary points of focus is feeling good and often any method in achieving it is promoted. Man was created as a feeling-based being. However, after the fall, feelings took center stage. They were a by-product of thoughts and desires opposed to God. Such is the reality of life in the physical world in a sin-cursed body. Sin, misery, and death entered the world after Adam's sin and God's judgment (Romans 5:12-14). Only the believer had been changed from the inside out. Only the believer can think God's thoughts, desire what God desires, and function as a God-pleaser. Therefore, the Bible calls men to think and desire according to biblical truth with the motivation to please God. To the degree that a person is motivated to please God, feelings will not be a person's guide to thoughts, desires, or actions. Rather the believer will imitate Jesus Christ who thought God's thoughts and desired what God desired. God-pleasing actions followed.

Further, there is the prevailing idea in culture that it is good and desirable to stay healthy, to have a well-functioning body, to have a prolonged life, and to avoid death. As we have already discussed those desires may or may not be wrong. A potential good desire becomes wrong when it takes center stage in one's life, thereby controlling the person's thinking, desiring, and acting. Those desires are inordinate when they are done apart from trusting God in His providence including giving the believer the body that he or she has. When feelings rule, relief becomes the goal rather than pleasing God.

So, you see that there are many things to consider in being a patient. Being a patient is a theological activity and being a God-honoring patient requires correct theology.

This book is designed to help you develop that theology and enjoy applying it.

CHAPTER 3

Specifics of Why Go To The Doctor: Biblical Stewardship

THIS SECTION CONSIDERS THE SPECIFICS of "why go to the doctor." The Bible gives three reasons for seeking medical. They are:

1. Biblical stewardship;
2. The creational fact that man is a whole person, a unit: body and soul or heart;
3. The relationship between the physical—outer—and the spiritual—inner man.

Each reason is important. It is helpful to compare these reasons with those normally given for seeking medical help. We will discuss each topic individually in successive chapters beginning with stewardship in this chapter.

Stewardship is a biblical concept that differs markedly from the culture's definition. Today, in response to the word steward, a person may think of an airline hostess or someone who seats you at a restaurant. In Biblical times, a steward was a servant who was entrusted to manage his master's household in his absence and then he was to give an account of his stewardship on the master's return.

A simple definition for biblical stewardship is taking care of that which God has entrusted to the believer. Since everyone is a steward (good or bad) and taking care of one's body is included in stewardship, going to the physician is relevant to our discussion of stewardship. Stewardship involves God-given responsibility, with accountability (Luke 16:1-13; 19:11-27; Matthew 25:14-30).

The Christian is a steward because he is united to Christ and in fellowship with Him. One of the words God has chosen to describe the Christian is steward (1 Corinthians 4:2). The believer has been entrusted with resources including his body. The key is being faithful in the exercise of that stewardship. The issue for every believer is this: will you be a good or a poor steward? The kind of steward a person is grows out of their view of their relationship with Christ and how important they consider that relationship to be. Wrong thinking about God, self, and our bodies leads us to wrong thinking and actions about all of life including stewardship of the whole person. A good steward is one who lives faithfully indebted to their trustworthy God

Further, stewardship involves taking care of the body which in God's providence has been given to the believer irrespective of whether it is failing or not. The issue is not the body that we have but taking care of that which God has entrusted to us.

What does stewardship have to do with taking care of our body? The body we have is the only one we will get in this life. God shows concern for our body and He has written instructions that deal with its care. Consider Paul's words in 1 Corinthians 6:12-20:

"Everything is permissible for me"—but not everything is beneficial. "Everything is permissible for me"—but I will not be mastered by anything. "Food for the stomach and the stomach for food"—but God will destroy them both. The body is not meant for sexual immorality, but for the Lord, and the Lord for the body. By his power God raised the Lord from the dead, and he will raise us also. Do you not know that your bodies are members of Christ himself? Shall I then take the members of Christ and unite them with a prostitute? Never! Do you not know that he who unites himself with a prostitute is one with her in body? For it is said, "The two will become one flesh." But he who unites himself with the Lord is one with him in spirit. Flee from sexual immorality. All others sins a man commits are outside his body, but he who sins sexually sins against his own body. Do you not know that your body is a temple of the Holy Spirit, who is in you, whom you have received from God? You are not your own; you were bought at a price. Therefore honor God with your body.

Paul taught that God designed the body and therefore He has something to say about its use and care. One's body is not for self pleasure (in these verses the context is sexual immorality, but Paul's words have a much broader context). One's body is to be used in the service of the Lord within the body of Christ. Good stewardship of the body is one way of serving the Lord, and faithfully serving the Lord is good stewardship. In these verses, Paul spells out important truths of good stewardship:

1. The body is the Lord's—it is not yours: verses 19-20;

2. The Lord is for the believer and his body: verse 14;

3. The bodily resurrection of Christ and that which God promised to the believer is God's guarantee that God is for the body: verse 14. Therefore, the believer is to be for the body God's way;

4. The individual believer is part of the larger body of Christ (the church): verse 15. What affects one, affects all members of the body of Christ;

5. The believer is indwelt by the Holy Spirit: verse 19;

6. The believer's body is not his—it is the Lord's and is to be used for glorifying Him in building up His church as the believer grows in Christlikeness: verse 20.

Paul taught that God has much invested in the believer who has been bought with a price (v.20). The believer is the Lord's—body and soul, inner (heart) and outer (body) man. Therefore, the Christian has no logical choice except to please God in and with his body. Good stewardship is the believer's only reasonable act of daily worship (Romans 12:1-2). Taking care of one's body in a God-honoring manner is fact and is not open for discussion.

Seeking medical help is one way in which to practice good stewardship. However, it should never be an end in itself. Good stewardship is seeking medical care for the purpose of pleasing God in a way that God requires and blesses regardless of the results (Matthew 6:33; 2 Corinthians 5:9,14-15). When a believer pleases God by being a good steward, he is living out God's original design as stated in Ephesians 1:4: "For he chose us in him before the creation of the world to be holy and blameless in his sight." Living according to God's original design is best for the believer, and it is the only way the believer can have a contented, simplified, satisfied life (Psalm 73:25-26; Matthew 11:28-30).

Please note that there are benefits of biblical stewardship. It is always to the believer's advantage to honor God in all that he does including being a patient. Consider some advantages of being a good steward. Pleasing God in terms of stewardship fulfills one of God's designs for man: man was designed in eternity past to be like Christ Who was the only person with Whom the Father was absolutely and ultimately well-pleased (Ephesians 1:4; Matthew 3:17; 17:5). Fulfilling God's design is the only way to live a satisfying and contented life. It is best for the believer and it honors God. When a person goes to the doctor in order to please Him, the person can, and should, rejoice even when the results are less than the person desired. God didn't promise to reverse the curse of sin in this life. That awaits resurrection. Until then, in this life failing bodies are a reality. However, when the believer is obedient to God's Word, God's promise of a blessed and simplified life is fulfilled (Matthew 11:28-30; Proverbs 3:5-8). This life may include healing and relief.

Another benefit centers on the release of us from the bondage of frantically seeking relief that may or may not happen. Obtaining relief may be a by-product of pleasing God through good stewardship but as I have pointed out previously, it is not guaranteed. Focusing on that which is impossible to obtain usually intensifies discomfort. And it doesn't please God. However, it is always possible for us to please God no matter the condition of our bodies. That truth should produce motivation, help, hope, and endurance as we respond to hard times God's way for God's glory. As a result, grumbling, complaining, and discontentment will be replaced by thankfulness, confidence, and reverence of a personal, sovereign, good God. Since pleasing God is the reason man was placed on this earth and the reason for salvation, functioning as a God-pleaser enables us to enjoy His relationship with God to the fullest as we anticipate heaven.

CHAPTER 4

Specifics of Why Go to the Doctor: Man as a Duplex Unit

A SECOND REASON FOR SEEKING medical care rests on the fact that man was created a duplex being (the term means two of something united). Man is a unit—a whole person. He is not simply body; he is not simply spirit. The Bible speaks of man's unity, duplexity, or wholeness when it refers to the material side of man which is the body (another term is outer person) and the immaterial side of a person (the inner person). Because man is a unit, good stewardship is concerned with the person's thoughts, desires, and actions. Feelings follow. Each of these activities occurs in the inner (heart) and outer person. This dual emphasis is a reflection of correct biblical anthropology (knowledge of mankind). It highlights God's original design of man and the fact that man is a whole person. Good stewardship requires proper knowledge and care of the spiritual and material side of man as a unit, a whole person.

The Bible describes the inner person by using several different terms. These include heart, mind, spirit, soul, will, and conscience. It is here that a person thinks, hopes, fears, purposes, doubts, considers, and decides on courses of action. This side of man never dies though the body is subject to death

(Romans 5:12-14; 2 Corinthians 4:16-18). It is important for every believer to remember the distinctive wholeness and unity of every person because the Bible teaches that man's body and its activity influences the inner person and inner-person activities affect the body

Based on these creational facts, it follows that biblical stewardship involves taking care of the whole person. Biblically speaking, the body includes the brain. The brain also goes into the ground and dies. There is no word for brain in the original language of the Bible (Greek or Hebrew language). From science we have learned that the brain functions as the receiver, integrator, and distributor of many body signals coming into it from the five senses (these include taste, touch, smell, hearing, and sight). In that sense, the brain is the control center of the body. The brain plays a role in determining how the body responds to various stimuli. Biblically the heart is man's control center. Scripture commands the believer to guard his heart which will affect his body (Proverbs 4:23). "For out of the overflow of the heart, the mouth speaks (Matthew 12:34; Mark 7:21).

Let's consider a few biblical "medical" facts. The Bible sets forth important truths about thinking and motivation. As mentioned above, the Bible teaches that people think, desire, and purpose in their inner person. The Bible, remember, distinguishes between a person's brain and the mind (another term for the inner you). In some way, not understood by science, but taught in the Bible, the inner and outer person are linked together so that each affects the other. Therefore, thinking and wanting occurs in both. As a result, the person develops habituated and patterned thinking and wanting and resultant actions. Feelings follow. These are reflections of the whole-person.

Science and practical living also tell us that thoughts and desires are interrelated and affect the way we feel and act. Biblically speaking, the issue is much deeper than mere scientific facts such as neurocircuitry, molecules, genes, and biochemistry. One's thought life and desires are also inner-man activities so that a person's thinking, wanting, doing, and feeling form an integral unit. Feelings and actions are connected to each other and flow out of a person's thoughts and desires. How a person feels affects what the person thinks, wants, and does or does not do; what a person does or does not do often affects feelings. Moreover, what a person thinks, and desires, influences feelings and actions. A summary of this biblical teaching is as follows: You feel what you feel because you do what you do and vice versa. And you feel what you feel because you think what you think; and you think what you think because you *want* what you want (You should read that over until you get it!).

To say that what is in a person's brain (or head) influences what they feel is not the same thing as saying that "it is all in your head." Rather, that which is going on in the inner person (heart) *and* the brain affects a person's feelings, thoughts, desires, and actions. These facts are important because a believer's inner person is the domain of the Holy Spirit and God's grace. It is not directly affected by disease and drugs.

When a believer changes his thinking or his desires for the good, it is the result of the Holy Spirit's work and not medications. What is the good? It is pleasing God as the believer becomes more like Christ by using the unpleasantness of life as a tool for imitating Christ. A metaphor for this concept of Christian growth is the Christian oyster (2 Corinthians 5:9). The oyster uses unpleasantness and irritation to make a pearl. The Christian uses unpleasantness to make the pearl of Christlikeness.

Modern medicine would have us believe that medications directly change thinking. Rather, people on drugs such as nerve pills and antidepressants report changed feelings. Drugs may change feelings in the body, and may even cloud thinking, but they never directly change thinking or motivation of the inner man. They are not the Holy Spirit.

The fact that the Bible speaks of the presence of and connection between inner- and outer-person activities can't be overemphasized. Modern culture doesn't understand or credit God for making man a duplex unit. But it indirectly acknowledges God's original design, when it utilizes varying techniques hoping to change and control a person's thinking with the sole goal of better feelings. Examples of these techniques include imagery, mindfulness, yoga, biofeedback, and distraction therapy. The phrase *mind over matter* is really misused because culture considers the mind and brain as the same.

Scripture describes the heart as the wellspring and source of life (Proverbs 4:23). The heart is the storehouse from which thoughts, attitude, affections/desires, actions, and motivations come. This biblical truth is expressed in Jesus' statement that man lives out of his heart (Matthew 15:8,16-20; Mark 7:20-23; Luke 6:43-45). Therefore, contrary to much medical teaching, it is critical to understand that the alleged changing of the brain and its chemistry through any number of resources (drugs and electroshock therapy for instance) doesn't change the heart/ inner man. The claim that it does ignores clear biblical teaching. In the believer, the heart is the fountain and wellspring of life and is the domain of the Holy Spirit (Proverbs 4:23; 14:27; 16:22). Contrary to scientific propaganda, man's moral compass isn't located in the brain. The Bible speaks of man's inner man using various terms such as heart, mind, soul, spirit, will, and conscience. Man was originally created morally-responsible as the image of the Creator. Sin didn't change God's original design. Man's morality resides in the inner man.

CHAPTER 5

Specifics of Why Go to the Doctor: The Relationship between the Physical and the Spiritual Aspects of Man

THE INTERACTION OF THE INNER-AND outer person is a third reason for properly seeking medical care. I have alluded to this fact in our previous discussion under man's duplexity. Inner-person activities such as what a person thinks and wants affect the body. In a similar manner, physical problems can result from as well as influence inner-person activities.

Medications and drugs do affect the body. A drug such as insulin in the diabetic may help control the person's glucose. Insulin is mandatory for the person with Type I diabetes because the insulin-producing cells are non-functioning. Insulin may be needed in patients with Type II diabetes, but oral medications are available. Adequately controlled blood sugars can help prevent subsequent complications. A drug may also affect the disease itself such as anticancer drugs or rheumatoid arthritis medication. All these examples focus on the effect of the drug on the body. In addition, a person's thinking may change for a variety of reasons as his physical problem is addressed and treated.

Let's consider the relationship of man's duplex unit from the physical (material) side. Bone fractures, arthritis, cancer, stroke, and heart disease are just some physical problems that people may face. Moreover, the brain and thinking may be affected directly (e.g.: a stroke) or indirectly (e.g.: a person's wrong focus on the failing body with its discomfort and unpleasantness). Outer-man failures hinder but do not cause inner-man responses. Please reread that sentence. It is true that physical problems can cause or contribute to an inefficiently functioning and diseased body. It is also true that wrong thinking and wanting lead to functional problems including complaints of fatigue, pain and stiffness, and abnormal thinking. The accompanying discomfort and the actual physical dysfunction from whatever cause can make it harder to think, desire, and act in a God-honoring manner.

We have learned that biblically speaking, physical problems are whole-person conditions so that the patient's thinking, fears, hopes, and expectations affect the person's response to the situation which is actually part of God's providential control of all things. Likewise, a damaged body can influence a person's thoughts and actions.

An interesting aspect of these biblical medical facts is evidenced in personal experience and what the culture and medical science call "positive thinking" and lifestyle changes. Positive thinking is encouraged in order to help a person produce better feelings and "cope" with his or her situation. However, the Bible teaches and exhorts the believer to think and desire according to biblical truth in order to please God which is what the believer was saved to do. Proper biblical thinking is never to be described as positive thinking. Rather, godly thinking and wanting influences a person's feelings and actions so that the believer "feels" better because he is! Conversely, ungodly thinking and wanting often aggravates and magnifies bad feelings (Proverbs 12:25; 14:30; 15:13, 30; 16:24; 17:22).

Biblical truth and its application always trump positive thinking because the believer's goal is primarily to please God and not simply please self. In addition, culture and medical science call for positive thinking and lifestyle changes but without a proper vertical reference. The Bible itself advocates so-called lifestyle changes but only those that flow from changed thinking and wanting that are part of the believer's growth in Christlikeness. We call them Christlikeness.

Some lifestyle changes include eating less and better, exercising more, and drinking certain beverages less and others more. These changes which can be part of good stewardship—if done only for relief or for better health miss the point of God's creational design for man and the Bible's dual emphasis on the inner and outer person. Biblical stewardship involves more than a positive attitude or lifestyle changes. A person doesn't need the Holy Spirit to make these changes. By definition, biblical stewardship means a change in a person's thinking about who they are, what they do, and Who God is and what He is doing. Biblical stewardship flows out of our relationship in Christ. Gratitude for Who God is and gratitude for salvation should motivate us, the believer to please God. Only the believer is motivated by love and gratitude for his Savior and the indwelling Holy Spirit. What follows will be a change in what we do with our bodies and the manner in which we do it.

CHAPTER 6
When Your Doctor Doesn't Have an Answer

AS I WROTE IN THE opening, going to the doctor is a part of American life. In some cases, the doctor may not be able to help you in the way you hoped. The doctor may diagnose you with an incurable disease or a chronic condition that may not respond to therapy. Or it may be that you have a condition that defies diagnosis or is terminal. Believer, how are you going to respond to such situations?

A major emphasis of this book has been to motivate every believer to seek medical attention for the right reasons. In order to accomplish this goal, the believer must recognize and act on the truth that going to the doctor is a theological activity. The application of biblical principles of stewardship is a key to functioning as a good theologian. To reiterate, biblical stewardship involves God-honoring thoughts, desires, and actions that address and flow from a heart that is focused on pleasing God.

Sometimes patients come to the doctor as good stewards, but the doctor really can't help them. Then what? Some would say pray and try to generate more faith. Yet many unbelievers are healed of various, even self-inflicted, ailments. They have no saving faith; so, is faith the answer? Yes and no. Rather, it is the faithful exercise of saving faith as an act of honor and respect to the God of the Bible.

Let me pause here to be clear about saving faith. I clarified "faith" by the adjective "saving" to highlight the truth that everyone has faith. Some have faith in their abilities, their money, their gifts, themselves, or their position. Some have faith in a God but view Him as someone who is obligated to give them healing. But saving faith has as its object the Triune God—Who He is and what He has done in Christ as applied by the Holy Spirit. Saving faith is the gift of God's saving grace by which a believer receives, rests, and relies upon the finished work of Christ Who died for His people in order to save them now and eternally.

It is of utmost importance for all believers to believe that resurrection and eternal life starts at the moment of salvation (John 17:3; Romans 6:9-10). After salvation, God grants enabling faith and sanctifying grace in order for the believer to grow more and more into the character of Christ.

The Bible has answers for all of life and especially in those instances where no physician has been able to make a difference in your medical condition. Consider the woman who had been bleeding for twelve years as described in Mark 5:24-34 (see parallel passages in Matthew 9:20-22; Luke 8:43-48).

> So Jesus went with him. A large crowd followed and pressed around him. And a woman was there who had been subject to bleeding for twelve years. She had suffered a great deal under the care of many doctors and had spent all she had, yet instead of get-

ting better she grew worse. When she heard about Jesus, she came up behind him in the crowed and touched his cloak, because she thought, "If I just touch his clothes, I will be healed." Immediately her bleeding stopped and she felt in her body that she was freed from her suffering. At once Jesus realized that power had gone out from him. He turned around in the crowd and asked, "Who touched my clothes?" "You see the people crowding against you," his disciples answered, "and yet you can ask, 'Who touched me?'" But Jesus kept looking around to see who had done it. Then the woman, knowing what had happened to her, came and fell at his feet and, trembling with fear, told him the whole truth. He said to her, "Daughter, your faith has healed you. Go in peace and be freed from your suffering."

Doctor Luke adds that the woman could not be healed by anyone (Luke 8:43-48). It is helpful to note the context of the miracle of the healing of the bleeding woman. In all three gospel accounts, Jesus was on His way to raise Jarius' daughter from the dead which He did (Matthew 9:18-19; Mark 5:21-24; Luke 8:40-42). Together, these two miracles continue the theme of Jesus as the Deliverer and Light of the world. He meets man's helplessness and despair in a dark world. Both the woman and Jarius sought Jesus out of a deep sense of impotence and waning hopefulness.

"But they found healing," you say. "What if I don't?" Today, the question for you and every believer is: what does it mean to seek Jesus with the body and condition that they have?

Should any person especially a believer seek "divine" healing? One aspect of seeking Jesus is developing and living out one's relationship with Christ. Paul spells out that truth in Philippians 3:3-11. In verses 3-6, Paul wrote that he was quite satisfied. As an unbeliever, he earnestly sought and valued himself. He lived for what he could get at that moment and the feelings that grew out of his performance. He did not seek Christ because Paul was Christ's enemy and he sought to kill Christ (John 15:18-21). After his conversion, there was a radical change in the object of Paul's allegiance. He sought a fuller and deeper intimacy with Christ (verses 7-11). He was consumed by God Himself; he was not concerned with getting things from God.

The term divine healing is not helpful. Here's why. All healing comes from the Lord—all healing is divine. It is easy to discount that fact and take for granted God's graciousness when there is improvement or cure in even the slightest abnormality. The mundane cures of colds just don't generate much interest in praising a healing God. The term divine healing is usually reserved for out-of-the-ordinary healings. However, both types of healing come from God to believers and unbelievers alike.

Returning to the gospel accounts, the woman had long-standing vaginal bleeding. The original word for her condition translated in verses 29 and 34 as trouble means scourging, whipping, or beating. [4] It is a powerful word indicating severe physical distress. Today, and perhaps then, we know that uncontrolled bleeding from any source can lead to anemia (low red blood cells due to iron deficiency) and fatigue. Perhaps abdominal and pelvic pain accompanied the bleeding. She

---

4. The term is used to describe Jesus' treatment at the hands of the Romans (Matthew 23:34; Luke 18:33; John 19:1).

was extremely uncomfortable. Her failing body was a burden. Earthly doctors had not provided relief. Over the course of twelve years, she had become impoverished physically and financially—by doctors! Moreover, she had lost her standing in society. By the very nature of her illness, she was considered ceremonially unclean (Leviticus 15:19-23). Her situation seemed hopeless.

Consider the medical scene at that time. The art of healing in Israel had several commendable features, especially when compared to the brand of medicine practiced by Gentile nations. Israelites believed in prayer to one God and in His healing effectiveness. Some knew that neither prayer nor faith heals; God does. The many regulations expressed in the laws of Israel, including the Ten Commandments, contributed to improved individual and public hygiene and better health. The laws of Israel addressed the whole person including both the mind and body. The Hebrew mindset contrasted for the dichotomy of the Greeks in terms of a person. The Hebrews considered man as a unit, body and inner person. The woman in Mark 5 had access to this high quality medical care and yet, in God's providence, treatments had been unsuccessful. Humanly speaking, her condition was incurable (Luke 8:43). Moreover, based on the prevalent theology, the woman would have been considered an unrepentant sinner deserving of her problem (see the book of Job; Luke 13:1-5; John 9:1-3). The lady had her physical problem and the burden of being shunned by her people.

Each gospel account accentuates one point: this miracle of healing points to Jesus as God Who came to rescue His people.

Access to Him is through saving faith expressed in action (Romans 5:2; Ephesians 2:18; 3:12). Helpless but not hopeless, after convincing herself that Jesus could heal her, the woman sought Him out (Mark 5:28). Several points of clarification are needed in order to understand the Lord's teaching. Otherwise, a person may make seeking Jesus for physical healing their major goal.

First, without saving faith it is impossible to please God (Hebrews 11:6). Again, I draw the distinction between saving and non-saving faith. Saving faith is given by God through the Holy Spirit; non-saving faith is generated by the person. The woman, out of desperation, expressed faith by going to doctors. Apparently, relief was her goal. Was she wrong or had she wasted her time in going to the doctors? No. She was not rebuked by Jesus for previous efforts to take care of her body. But in seeking Christ, she found the person Who heals not only the body but also the whole person—inside and out.

Initially, convinced of the power of Christ to heal, she sought to touch His garments (Mark 5:28). However, Jesus wasn't satisfied with simply healing her physically. He perfected her faith. He exposed her publicly, and with fear and trembling she responded (Mark 5:31-33). Face to face with Christ, her faith grew as she experienced God's person and power intimately. Saving faith is also enabling faith that moves a person to increasingly trust and depend on Jesus instead of self.

Second, the issue is never a matter of how *much* faith a person has. Rather, the issue is two-fold: firstly, whether one's faith is saving or non-saving faith; secondly, whether a person is fully faithful in expressing their faith. When the disciples complained that their faith was too small or that they lacked faith, Jesus rebuked them for their lack of faith or (more appropriately) their failure to faithfully trust and obey (Matthew 6:30; 8:26; 14:31; 16:8; 17:19-20; Luke 12:28; 17:5). By the words, "O you of little faith" Jesus confronted His doubting, fearful, bewildered, and even frantic disciples. Jesus made clear that the amount of faith is not basic. Rather, the solution to their problem (and every believer) is to trust and obey. How much faith a believer has is not the issue because saving faith is a gift from God and His gifts are never flawed in quality or quantity (Ephesians 2:8-9; James 1:17). The problem resides in the believer himself—he is to exercise the gift of faith. He does that by faithfully trusting in and holding on to God's promises and acting as if they are true—because they are (Romans 8:35-39; Hebrews 10:35-39; 11:1-3, 6). A lethargic believer whose faith is dormant or poorly developed should become an energetic believer through faithful and joyful obedience and application of God's truth to all of life. The blessing will come through the gift of saving faith when the person exercises that gift (John 13:17; James 1:25).

Jesus providentially placed His disciples in varying circumstances that demanded trust in God. His desire and goal was for them to become completely dependent, trusting people of the Triune God. The expression of the believer's faith is always growing, maturing, and increasing (1 Thessalonians 4:1-3; James 1:2-4; 1 Peter 1:6-10). Too often, believers function as men of little faith. Faithfulness increases, especially in tough times, as the Christian acts faithfully, expectantly, and joyfully upon the promises of God in His Word. It is so easy for every believer to live by feelings and the desire to have good ones. When that happens, the person's focus is self, and biblical truth is ignored.

We often say *forgotten* but I think that is a euphemism for failing to properly counsel ourselves. Later I will give various examples of growth in Christlikeness in times during which it seems and feels impossible to achieve

Third, Jesus' healing miracles testify to the truth that Jesus is God, the Healer and Deliverer. In Mark 5, the word translated healed in verses 28 and 34 is the Greek word *sozo* which means to save, to rescue, to deliver, or to heal. It always implies movement from some difficulty to its solution. It is used some fifty-four times in the Gospel accounts. Its use can be roughly divided as follows: fourteen times meaning to be saved from disease and demons; twenty times meaning to be rescued from death and peril; twenty times meaning spiritual salvation. In all three categories, *sozo* depicts the person being delivered from a seemingly hopeless condition. When saved from it, he finds security and refuge. When God saves, the person is rescued from bondage and darkness and is transferred to the kingdom of freedom and light (Colossians 1:13).

In using *sozo* the Holy Spirit brings together the spiritual and physical dimensions of life. Jesus came to seek and save those who were lost (Luke 19:10). He came to the sick and needy in contrast to those who did not think that they were spiritually sick (Matthew 9:12-13; Mark 2:17; Luke 5:30-31). The woman described in Mark 5 knew that she was sick and needy physically. It was not until her encounter with Jesus that she came to realize her "spiritual" neediness. Her awareness of her condition was in stark contrast to the ignorant arrogance of those who didn't think they needed a doctor. The growing awareness of her impotence led her to seek Christ. Finding Him provided insight into her need of complete dependence on God. She learned the futility of living apart from Him.

Finally, note that Jesus told the woman that it was her faith that brought healing (Mark 5:34). What did He mean? The phrase, your faith has healed you or made you well, occurs seven times in the Gospels: once in Matthew (9:22); twice in Mark (5:34; 10:52); and four times in Luke (7:50; 8:48; 17:19; 18:42). These seven occurrences involve four events: the bleeding woman, a blind man, a leper, and a sinful woman who had been forgiven much. All but one involves physical problems (See Luke 7:36-50 and Luke's account of a forgiven woman). Taken together these accounts help us understand that faith—in the abstract—doesn't save. It is the God of a believer's saving faith Who brings healing both physically and spiritually. The people described in each of the accounts described above grew as faithful, trusting, hopeful people. They were more impressed and thankful for their relationship to Christ than with the results of what Christ had done for them physically.

Look at the evidence of their growth. The blind man when asked by Jesus what he wanted replied, "that I may see again" (Mark 10:46-52; Luke 18: 35-43). Jesus clarified his expectations and then commanded him to see again. And he did! Then, in thankful reliance on Christ, he followed Jesus praising Him. The word translated followed (*akoloutheo*) is a relational word and indicates both a leaving and cleaving. Jesus had established a relationship with him. As a result, the blind man abandoned his former life for one of trust and obedient faith.

In like manner, one leper turned back from going the way Jesus had commanded and placed himself before Christ as an act of worship (Luke 17:16). Having received mercy, the cleansed leper purposefully and sensibly praised the One Who had been merciful. This Samaritan foreigner was the only one of the ten who returned to Jesus because only he truly understood the significance of his physical cleansing. Jesus said that this man knew what it meant to put saving faith in action while the others did not.

And in Luke 7:50, the woman who had been forgiven much also recognized her great need for forgiveness and the Forgiver. She demonstrated that understanding by personally serving Christ. Her response was in stark contrast to Simon the Pharisee who had failed to supply Jesus and his guests with water as a common courtesy (Luke 7:44-47). In humble, informed, and repentant faith, she drew closer to Jesus whereas Simon distanced himself.

Reader, how do you respond to these accounts? Do you say, "Great for them, but what about me? I have come to Jesus in prayer and hope, but He doesn't answer me with healing. All these people were healed. No wonder they were grateful. What about those of us who don't get healed? What are we to be grateful for?"

Physical healing and relief may come as result of prayer and being a good steward. However, and I repeat, God makes no such guarantee. Rather, what God does guarantee is growth in grace and Christlikeness, which is the best thing this side of heaven (Philippians 2:12-13). It is what believers were designed to do; it is complete freedom; and it is the only resource for living a satisfied and contented life irrespective of problems, physical or otherwise (Ephesians 1:4; Matthew 11:28-30).

In God's providence, the believer's growth is achieved most noticeably and effectively in tough times, including physical problems. Satisfaction comes from pleasing God rather than getting relief but only when the believer's focus is on becoming more like Christ.

The woman in Mark 5 went away healed physically, but what she had learned spiritually was far greater. In verse 34, Jesus' words to her must have been as a soothing balm to her ravaged body and her anguished thoughts: "Daughter, your faith has healed you. Go in peace and be freed from your suffering."

Jesus called this woman who was probably about His age or older "Daughter" denoting that she was His Child. She may have been a babe in the faith, but she was His! What comfort and tenderness He expressed! He praised her faith, or better, the faithful exercise of it. He made it a point to show her His response to her faith. She had been healed physically before talking to Jesus face to face. Now she was beginning to understand that physical healing pointed her to complete dependence on God through Jesus. Initially she moved toward Jesus seeking physical help. In reality, she found Christ after He had found her! Christ exhorted her to rejoice and live as a one who had been released from bondage though His goodness and power (Mark 5:34). Such is God's lesson for all believers.

"All great," you respond, "but how does failure to heal me help me to express trust, gratitude, and dependence on God?" This is a very good questions that deserves a very good answer.

If we as believers seek after Christ to get physical healing only, we have missed the point of Jesus' teaching. We must function from the perspective that our physical condition creates a context for demonstrating faithful trust and dependence on Christ irrespective of the success or failure of medical treatment. The physical condition is one context in which we are to develop the attitude expressed by David and Paul: they could not get enough of the Triune God (Psalm 34:8; 2 Corinthians 12:7-10; Philippians 3:7-11). So how do you move closer to Jesus when your body is failing, and medical treatment has not produced the desired results? In other words, what does it mean to go to Jesus and how will that look (Matthew 11:28-30)?

First, you must come to understand and act upon the truth that God has not reversed the effects of the curse of sin. Deteriorating and decaying bodies are part of that curse. So, too, is the failure of medical science and treatment. So where does that leave you? It forces you back to the Bible. And your relationship with Christ by the Holy Spirit (2 Corinthians 12:7-10). As we have just learned, Jesus taught that hurting bodies are uncomfortable realities for everyone and are reminders of God's judgment upon mankind. Jesus was soon to become an expert in this area (Isaiah 53). The cross testifies to that fact—it took the cross and the shed blood of Christ to redeem believers from the curse. Rather, rightly understood, failing bodies also demonstrate the believer's dependent position in God's universe, and their need for Christ. That is a fundamental biblical truth that is often neglected and even scorned. Without a proper understanding of these truths even the believer will use whatever means that is available in order to get what they have deemed best for them—relief and physical healing. The person may even try Jesus in order to get it.

Second, recognize that the fundamental need for and in life is not physical (Luke 10:38-42). Praying to Jesus is God's means for every believer to fellowship with God and to communicate hopes and desires. But it is more than that. Prayer is one of God's ways for God's people in every situation to express hope and dependence on Him. God created every person a dependent being, and prayer expresses that dependency. Before salvation, the believer had a much bigger problem than a failing body or maintaining good health. As demonstrated by the woman in Mark 5, every person needs a heart change. Before salvation every person was God's enemy, an outlaw, a rebel, and a renegade desiring nothing to do with Him. Now, believer, your greatest need and privilege is becoming more like the Savior in thought, desire, and action. Unless we grasp this truth and relish its significance, we will be tossed back and forth in a sea of misery and sadness (James 1:8; 4:8). As you develop Christlikeness daily using what God gives in His providence (including unpleasantness), God is glorified, and your life is simplified. Please remember that the only way possible to please God is to become more like His Son in Whom God was perfectly and completely well pleased. I repeat: becoming more like Christ includes using every situation to think, desire, and act more like Him. What awaits us as believers on Judgment is God's pronouncement: well done good and faithful servant enter into my kingdom (Matthew 25 and Luke 19). These words must have been spoken to Jesus as He ascended to heaven (Hebrews 12:1-3).

Third, as good as having a healthy body may be, it pales when we truly consider a fundamental aspect of life which is growing, changing, and becoming more like Christ (2 Corinthians 12:7-10). God prepares us for heaven by placing us in situations that are beyond our control. In that way, we are forced to look away from self and to focus upward and outward thereby imitating Christ (Hebrews 12:1-3). We are to live well in every situation even when feelings and the culture shout to us otherwise. We are to live well, in part, so that we will die well. We await and long for our resurrected body and being in the very presence of the great and awesome Triune God (1 John 3:1-3). However, we are not home yet. Heaven awaits but so does living in God's world for His glory with physical or presumed physical problems. By looking forward and outward we have a foretaste of heaven. Unless you, believer, have that perspective, you will give up, give in, and/or grumble and complain (Numbers 11, 21; Philippians 2:14-17). In fact, too often believers function as the unbeliever and live the lie. We are tempted to foolishly and arrogant attempt to seize control from God by attempting to get out of the situation through relief. Rather God's way is to rely on His powerful, good control and grow in Christlikeness (1 Corinthians 10:13). That pleases God and is best for us.

Coming to Jesus means perceiving life from an eternal perspective. It is possible to live this earthly life as if heaven was a bad place. Too often fascination with this life and the mindset of the culture results in an earthly-mindedness. Having things "my" way takes precedent, and the desire to get it can dominate a person's life. When that happens, the person fails to consider and apply a major lesson of the cross: using what is bad and disliked for good. In the case of failing physical health, or the desire for good health, believers are to use what they don't like or wish they had to become more like Christ, which, I repeat, is the most important activity for any believer while on this earth.

Rightfully understood, coming to Jesus is as applicable today as it was in Jesus' day. The proper motivation for coming to Jesus is to honor God rather than to get better feelings, relief, and or healing. Those may come but as by-products of good stewardship. The proper way to come to Jesus is to first acknowledge who He is and what He has done for us. The practice of good stewardship will follow out of dependent and humble thankfulness for our relationship with our Savior. Learn and follow what the psalmist wrote in Psalm 73:25-26:

> Whom have I in heaven but you? And earth has nothing I desire besides you. My flesh and my heart may fail, but God is the strength of my heart and my portion forever.

CHAPTER 7

When God Says
No to Healing

THE BIBLE HIGHLIGHTS THE FACT that every person's body will fail, sometimes sooner than later, with death as the ultimate failure (Romans 5:12-14; 2 Corinthians 4:16-18). That is the reality of living in a fallen world. Bodies sometimes fail to improve despite treatment that has proven effective in other patients with the same physical condition. What is a person to think about these truths? How is he to respond to such failure?

The initial reaction is to consult with the medical community for relief. While not wrong, please remember that the desire for a changed body must never be the Christian's driving force for seeking help. God has something better for you and every Christian. Christ's resurrected body alone sets the norm. The reality of a normally functioning body awaits heaven (1 Corinthians 15:42-49, 56; 2 Corinthians 5:1-9). God perfects His people in a variety of ways. One means of accomplishing growth in Christlikeness is the reality of failing bodies. Failing bodies are the result of God's judgment on Adam and Eve in the Garden. However, God did not leave His people to fend for themselves. God equips and exhorts them to learn one of the lessons of the cross: hard times are to be approached and responded to as an opportunity to imitate Christ by focusing on pleasing God (2 Corinthian 12:7-10). This may seem impossible when faced with unpleasantness and uncertainty. At times the situation and condition may seem as if the person is in a hole too deep, on a mountain too high, or in a tunnel so long that there is no hope. Biblical truth meets the believer, a child of the Father and of the King, where he is, and helps him reevaluate himself and the situation. The believer then functions in a God-honoring manner which brings joy and gratitude in the situation and not necessarily out of it (1 Corinthians 10:13).

The first truth to remember and apply whenever healing hasn't come is that this is God's world. He directs and sustains His people and their actions because He is the good and merciful Creator, Owner, Originator, Sustainer, Provider, and Ruler. Therefore, what comes to every believer comes from His wise and loving hand. What God sovereignly ordains is for His glory and the benefit of His people. What benefits His people the most, as we have seen, is for them to grow in Christlikeness. Sometimes He does that by saying no to healing (2 Corinthians 12:7-10; James 1:2-4; 1 Peter 1:6-7).

The second truth to remember and apply is that since failing health is part of living in a sin-cursed, fallen world, responding to it is an ever-present obligation and privilege in this life. Ask yourself, how do you respond to your failing body and to God's no to your prayer for relief?

The third truth to remember and apply is that a response to God's providence is a response to God! Complaints about providential happenings (whether it is the weather, your body, or another person) are complaints against God.

A fourth truth centers on the fact that seeking relief is not necessarily wrong. However, seeking relief becomes wrong when the focus is on what we want rather than on growth in Christlikeness. God wants us to be a good steward not only of our body but of adverse situations as well. God intends for us to use what we don't like to become more like His Son Who was the only Person in Whom God was truly and completed.

These truths are exemplified by Paul, a man of sorrows (2 Corinthians 4:8-10; 6:4-10; 11:23-28; 12:7-10). After reading the accounts of God's providence in his life including his physical condition, you might think that Paul would have given up or tried harder to control things. But he says just the opposite in 2 Corinthians 1:8-10.

> We do not want you to be uninformed, brothers, about the hardships we suffered in the province of Asia. We were under great pressure, far beyond our ability to endure, so that we despaired even of life. Indeed, in our hearts we felt the sentence of death. But this happened that we might not rely on ourselves but on God, who raises the dead. He has delivered us from such a deadly peril, and he will deliver us. On him we have set our hope that he will continue to deliver us.

He and the brothers were in a tight squeeze. Humanly speaking it looked like death was to be the only outcome for them. Yet God delivered them for at least one purpose: to help them develop a growing reliance and trust in God rather than on themselves (v.9). He learned this lesson well as we read in 2 Corinthians 4:8-10.

> We are hard pressed on every side, but not crushed;
> perplexed, but not in despair; persecuted, but not
> abandoned; struck down, but not destroyed. We
> always carry around in our body the death of Jesus,
> so that the life of Jesus may also be revealed in
> our body.

Paul wrote that he was down, but he was not out. Humanly speaking, things were bleak. Paul had encountered a myriad of circumstances all of which took a toll on his body. Yet, he stayed the course and fought the good fight (1 Timothy 1:18; 4:6-7; 2 Timothy 2:5; 4:7). That fight didn't include coping, accepting, or tolerating his condition. Rather, he made it his goal and ambition to please God using his failing body as the platform on which to do so (2 Corinthians 5:9). But Paul was no stoic. He hurt and he acknowledged it. Paul even cried out to God for relief and healing, and he wasn't wrong for doing so.

> To keep me from becoming conceited because of
> these surpassingly great revelations, there was given
> me a thorn in my flesh, a messenger of Satan, to
> torment me. Three times I pleaded with the Lord
> to take it away from me. But he said to me, "My
> grace is sufficient for you, for my power is made
> perfect in weakness." Therefore I will boast all the
> more gladly about my weaknesses, so that Christ's
> power may rest on me. That is why, for Christ's sake,
> I delight in weaknesses, in insults, in hardships, in
> persecutions, in difficulties. For when I am weak,
> then I am strong.

In these verses the Holy Spirit affirms powerful, transforming truths especially with reference to God's providence and physical problems. In 2 Corinthians 12:1-6, Paul wrote that he had visions and revelations. In response, God sent a physical malady as a means of humbling him (verse 7). Imagine that. Paul had not asked for those revelations but in response to God's activity God purposefully brought a physical problem to bear on Paul.

Paul acknowledged God's sovereign power and control and Satan as God's agent (many think this problem was eye related: Galatians 4:13-15; 6:11). He sought relief by going to God in prayer pleading with Him three times (verse 8). Verse 9 records God's resounding no. One can only wonder at Paul's initial thinking. In contrast to Paul's response in verse 10, it might be easy to say such things as: "How can God do this to me. I have kingdom work to do. I am a first-class missionary with places to go and people to save" Or, "I don't have time to slow down."

God's no is startling enough but His explanation is even more so: "My grace/help is sufficient for you." The word "sufficient" carries with it the idea of enough, contentment, and satisfaction. In John 14:8-9, Philip using the same word, asked Jesus to show them the Father and that would be enough. Jesus answered by saying He is the *Enough*: if you have seen Me you have seen the Father. Jesus taught Philip the same lesson as the Holy Spirit taught Paul but not in the context of physical problems. In other words, God told Paul that he needed nothing more than the grace that comes through a relationship with Him. Having a relationship with God in Christ, and receiving God's grace, is far more important than relief. In fact, God's no is testimony to that fact. So I ask: how are you handling

God's "no"? The answer is of fundamental importance to you and for you.

The Holy Spirit was making clear that not all sickness is removed by prayer—some is removed without prayer (unbelievers are healed). Some people are never relieved of their problems physical or otherwise. Through the providence of non-healing, Paul learned that sickness does have a beneficial purpose. He learned that it is never the bad times or sickness per say but his response that is key. In verse 10, Paul's response makes clear that he is a good student and that he has learned God's lesson well.

So far, we have discussed God's response to giving Paul revelations, Paul's prayer for relief, and God's "no." Each response unfolds the ever-increasing depth of God's wisdom, goodness, and power. Each response was startling in its own right. What follows from the pen of Paul is nothing less than amazing: Paul gratefully glories in his weakness! He prayed that God would bring any and every circumstance that limited or removed his ability to control them because he knew that growing and changing in Christlikeness was God's best for him. He knew that times of trouble facilitated growth. Contentment and sufficiency came in his afflictions, because, in them, he depended on God rather than self. When he did, he grew and changed into Christlikeness. Paul's contentment is evidence of his growth as he imitated Christ (Philippians 4:10-13; John 4:31-34; 5:19-30). Since Paul's contentment came from his relationship with Christ, Paul would not detract from that dependency.

So, reader, go to God in prayer and ask, even plead, with Him for relief as an act of humble dependency. But look beyond the relief. Real relief in this life is not simply lack of physical problems or good health. What is important is to be what God designed you to be—a person after His own heart who desires to become like Jesus Christ. These exhortations are countercultural and counterintuitive. So often, we think in terms of getting for self by self and to self. The Bible sets forth an agenda that flows from a radically different mindset and lifestyle only in the believer.

We are to learn the lesson that the Holy Spirit is teaching us through Paul. Genuine relief of the whole person awaits heaven, but it begins here on this earth. It may include physical relief. However, genuine relief comes despite physical healing and often comes as a result of God's no. Pleasing the Father is what motivated Jesus throughout His life (John 4:31-34; 17:1-5). When our desire is to please Him and develop Christlikeness, like Paul and like Christ, we will use whatever affliction, physical or otherwise, to develop a greater dependency on God in Christ. God's no to healing should lead to a greater appreciation of Christ, what you are in Christ, and a more fruitful ministry for His great Name. If it hasn't, ask yourself why not and then reread this chapter of the book to help you become more like Christ.

How Should a Patient Relate to a Physician?

HAVING DISCUSSED THREE BIBLICAL REASONS for seeking medical care, the next order of business is to consider what a patient is to think and do when he goes to the physician. Based on the information given in the previous section, I have established that every believer is to receive medical care as a good theologian by functioning as God's kind of steward. In this way we honor God and reap the benefits of pleasing God.

What are we to think and do when we see the doctor? We will answer those questions using five categories:

1. We are to function as a good theologian. All of life is theological and everyone is a theologian because everyone has a belief about God and is in or out of proper relationship with Him;

2. We are to function as a planner: every patient should develop goals and a plan to achieve them;

3. We are to function as a listener: in order to learn;

4. We are to function as an inquirer: you should gather sufficient facts through listening in order to interpret them adequately;

71

5. We are to function as an implementer. As a good theo-logian-steward, you are to apply what you have learned in the office, and perhaps outside of it, depending on your reading activities regarding the problem.

CHAPTER 8

Important Biblical Truths

ABOVE ALL, REMEMBER THAT ALL of life is theological, and that everyone is a theologian. What I don't mean by the term "theologian" is one who studies theological books (though that activity is not wrong and theological study is of much benefit). Rather, I mean that everyone looks at life through God's truth as taught in the Bible or through some other source of professed truth such as one's feelings, reasoning, experience, observations, or medical science. A good theologian is one whose view of God is derived from the Bible and correctly impacts the person's thinking, wanting, and acting in every situation of life. A good theologian relies on one standard—biblical truth—and moves out into other areas. He does not begin with facts derived by using some other standard. These truths are crucial to developing "good theology." An atheist is a theologian but a poor one. He denies the existence of God and lives contrary to God. Yet God affects his life!

Since these two truths (life is theological and everyone is a theologian) are foundational to being God's kind of patient, we need to understand the Bible's teaching on this subject. These truths are written over all the pages of Scripture beginning in Genesis 1-2. From this portion of Scripture, we learn that man was created after God's image rather than *after their own kind* as God created the animals (Genesis 1:11-12, 21, 24-25; 26-28). Not only was man created after a divine pattern, God formed man in an entirely different manner. He breathed the breath of life into him (*the Lord God formed a man from the dust of the ground and breathed into his nostrils the breath of life, and the man became a living being.* Genesis 2:7).

God placed man in the Garden for a specific purpose: to work and take care of it (literally guard it). Man was a theologian and steward from the very beginning (Genesis 2:15). God did not leave man to his own devices and thoughts. Adam was not autonomous. He was a revelation receiver. He was designed to receive counsel and direction from outside of himself. He was dependent on this counsel for living joyously, purposely, and productively in God's world. God blessed Adam and Eve and He gave them specific instructions: *Be fruitful and increase in number; fill the earth,subdue it, and rule over it* (Genesis 1:28). In addition, God expected man to interpret His revelation in light of His word. Adam and Eve were given instructions in the form of general principles, except for the specific injunction not to eat from the tree of knowledge of good and evil (Genesis 1:28; 2:15-17). Apart from that command, they had liberty and ability to consider how best to implement (apply) God's orders.

In the Garden before sin, Adam and Eve were in perfect relationship to God, His created world, and to each other. The reason: God was in perfect relationship to them. They personally walked with God Who reminded them of their dependence on Him. Not only was God omnipresent but Adam and Eve acknowledged, embraced, and enjoyed God's presence. Being in relationship with God was to control all that Adam and Eve did as they fulfilled his covenant responsibilities by obeying God's orders (Genesis 1:28; Romans 5:12-15; 1 Corinthians 15:45)

Further, as covenantal head of mankind and as an individual, Adam's relationship to God required him to function as a God-pleaser. Adam was created a morally responsible being. Adam's relationship to God was an ethical one. Adam was in a proper relationship with God. He was to respond to God's revelation with undivided loyalty, allegiance, and devotion and lead Eve in that activity. Pleasing God was in their best interest.

What was true and best for pre-fall Adam and Eve remains true and best for every person today. Everyone is either in or out of relationship to God the Creator. Everyone owes loyalty, allegiance, and devotion to God and still needs to receive revelation from God. However, because of sin and man's sinfulness, revelation is no longer given as it was given to Adam. Truth is now found in the Bible. Everyone is to understand, interpret, and apply (implement) that truth in all areas of life—including taking care of the body. However, sin and God's judgment changed man and man's relationship to God. Mankind began to function according to the manifesto of: for me, by me, and to me. Self took center stage.

Post-fall, mankind's condition is not a pretty picture. However, Paul sums up the graciousness, love, mercy, and righteousness of God in several places in Scripture with "but now": (Romans 3:21; Ephesians 2:4). God stepped in as only He can. Unless a person is regenerated, he can't and won't think God's thoughts, desire God's desires, and act according to God's revealed will. Being a Christian compels both the patient and physician to receive, accept, and practice biblical truth for God's glory and the good of His church and individual believers.

CHAPTER 9

Application: Being a
Patient God's Way

WE HAVE STUDIED THE BIBLE'S teaching that the basis for
life is theological and everyone is a theologian. Now we are
ready to discuss how to apply these truths. Being a good theologian is the essence of being a faithful steward. In terms of
receiving medical care, being a good theologian means several
things. First it means receiving information from the doctor
or other health care provider. There may be other sources
of information, but in our culture, doctors are considered
knowledgeable in the area of health care. However, none of
these sources is to be equated with biblical revelation. Second,
it means evaluating information according to biblical truth
in order to understand the truth of its content and implications. Interpreting information must be in light of God's word.
Having done so, the good theologian will apply what he has
learned according to Scripture in a way that glorifies God and
benefits the person.

Let me explain more fully. Medical care is relational. The
Bible focuses on relationships beginning with the Trinity in
eternity past, extending to God's relationship with every person, and human personal relationships. Medical care involves
several relationships: the patient-doctor relationship and the

relationship of both to God—whether these are acknowledged or not. The proper application of biblical principles of stewardship by you, (the receiver), and the doctor, (the giver), enables the believer to function as a good theologian. In the giving and receiving of medical care, a bad theologian fails to acknowledge both the patient's and the doctor's relationship to God. This is a critical point!

Others, besides medical practitioners, recognize that the human relationship (man to man) is crucial for the practice of "good" medicine. In medical school, physicians are taught to interact well (positively) with patients. A term for this interaction is popularly called "bedside manner." However, the doctor isn't the principle party in the relationship; it is God. To the degree that a patient's or doctor's relationship to the God of the Bible is not represented in some form, God is ignored. When that happens, going to the doctor becomes functional atheism.

Your relationship to Christ may be further avoided, distorted, or given token acknowledgement by the addition of the vague and abstract term spirituality. Some Christians are taken in by such talk and are led astray—because they are not good theologians. The Bible focuses on a proper understanding of spirituality. Certain segments of the medical community and the culture agree that spirituality is vital to good patient care. However, they don't agree with the Bible's definition of it. Nonbiblical definitions of spirituality abound but underlying all of them is self. In contrast, the Bible refers to "biblical spirituality." This term is not found in the Bible, but by it I am referring to the indwelling of the Holy Spirit in the believer and in the Church (1 Corinthians 3:16-17 and 6:19; 2 Corinthians 6:14-7:1). God desires and equips the believer and the Church with the

Word and the Spirit so that the believer and the Church thinks God's thoughts, desires what God desires, and acts according to biblical truth. Energized and motivated by the Holy Spirit, the believer, patient and doctor, will bring their thinking, wanting, and actions in line with biblical truth.

Reader, consider ways that you and others may function apart from such a relationship to Christ. A few illustrations will help you examine yourself in this area. You may view the doctor as someone who is to "make" you feel better no matter the cost. Or you may view him as a body mechanic expecting him to keep you going. You may uncritically accept lifestyle and behavioral changes suggested by your doctor without reference to your relationship to Christ as efforts to gain or maintain good health. Any of these approaches are warnings that you be may be forgetting and actually jettisoning the practice of biblical stewardship.

In order for any believer to function as a good steward, we must think vertically as a whole person. One of life's goals is pleasing God with the body that He has given us. There is one great Healer, Savior, and Deliverer and He has returned to heaven. Taking care of your body and receiving healing is not the same thing. In the end, serving God is the best thing that you can do to remain healthy. And since pleasing God through serving Him is to be your goal, awaiting Christ's final healing will not be a burden. Rather using the failing body to please Him now becomes a blessed adventure as we rely on His grace (Galatians 2:20; Philippians 4:13).

There are some who have lost sight of the fact that good medicine is relational. Therefore, the patient-physician relationship is under fire. Patients are inundated with filling out forms in place of interacting with doctors and nurses. Patients are encouraged to speak about what ails them in highly specific terms while the whole person is ignored, or the patient is sent to some mental health worker. Physicians—as persons—are viewed as expendable parts of the medical care system and are only deliverers of a product called medical care. Time spent with patients is often consumed with checking boxes and is limited for the sake of so-called productivity.

It is in this climate of secularism and big business that believers, both patient and physician, are called by God to focus on being good stewards by bringing their relationship to Christ to bear on the receiving and giving of medical care. That isn't easy; often pressure to the contrary may be brought to bear on both parties. The temptation to leave behind their relationship to Christ can be overwhelming. This book is designed to help you faithfully practice biblical stewardship no matter the situation.

CHAPTER 10

The Patient as a Goal-Maker and Planner

AN IMPORTANT ASPECT OF FUNCTIONING as God's kind of patient involves coming to the doctor and the plan for implementing good stewardship principles. Life is characterized by making choices, setting goals, and pursuing them. I repeat: our goal as believers is to please God rather than pleasing ourselves (2 Corinthians 5:9, 14-15). When seeking medical care, all other goals must be subordinate to this primary goal. When other goals become the driving force, we fail to honor God. Some of these goals include maintaining good health, prolonging life, finding relief for physical problems, coping, getting by, looking good to others, and avoiding death.

Let's be clear about this. Some of the goals listed above may not be wrong in themselves. However, when any of them become the driving force in our lives, functionally they become more important than our desire to please God. When that happens, we have placed our desire for relief above honoring God and being a good steward. The Bible calls this changed status of a desire a direct attack on God and idolatry (Ephesians 5:5; Colossians 3:5).

As I have noted, the Bible teaches that everyone lives out of his heart (Matthew 6:19-24; Luke 12:34-36). Think for a moment: where is your treasure? Where your heart and treasure are defines your goal and motivation. Your treasure is what you seek after, desire, live for, and must have. These things define you! Seeking after something for self is directly opposed to Jesus' summary of life in Matthew 22:37-40. Loving God and loving one's neighbor is to be the major life focus of every believer. It is not loving self. Loving self is already part of the problem. The phrase is a misnomer because it reflects self-absorption and self-exaltation. If loving self was to be the believer's main focus, getting relief would never compete with being a good steward of the body.

In my experience, it is not uncommon for patients to come to the office with a "want list" spelling out their hopes and desires. Included in the list are such desires as remaining in the best health possible, relief, and the hope that whatever they have can be treated and improved. Each patient has wants and goals. A key factor in functioning as a good steward is to rethink goals and desires before going to the doctor.

Moreover, since no one on this earth can outrun the effects of the curse of sin upon the body, going to the doctor primarily for the reasons stated in the "want list" will be futile and unsuccessful (Romans 5;12-14; 2 Corinthians 4:16-18). There is only One who is the Divine Healer. Jesus has promised upon His return to restore all life. He is the Life-giving Spirit because He is Life (1 Corinthians 15:45; John 5:26; 14:6). This restoration includes resurrection in a glorified body (1 Corinthians 15:42-49). As I have written, God has not chosen to completely reverse the effect of the curse of sin on the body in this life. That awaits the believer's entrance into heaven. In this present life God expects us to apply biblical principles as a good steward as we progress in Christlikeness. Every time we deviate from that biblical agenda, we will seek that which God has not promised on this earth. This seeking leads only to dissatisfaction, futility, and bondage. What foolishness!

CHAPTER 11

The Patient as a Listener and Learner

A SECOND ACTIVITY THAT IS crucial for functioning as God's kind of patient is to be a listener for the purpose of learning. Biblical listening is an aspect of good stewardship. Listen as a learner and then process the information that you receive through the use of biblical principles. Developing a learner's spirit is one means of developing Christlikeness. It is becoming more like Christ because Jesus Himself learned obedience (Hebrews 2:10; 5:8). The disciples (as their name means) were students. Jesus took them with Him in order to help them become like Him (Mark 3:14; Luke 6:40; Acts 4:13). Likewise, believers are called to imitate Christ (1 Corinthians 11:1; 1 Peter 2:21; 3 John 11). Therefore, you should be willing to hear the medical data about you and the doctor's interpretation of it. Listening carefully to learn in order to evaluate what you hear requires a humble spirit and wise heart.

Assuming the role of a learner might require silence as you listen. That may be hard, but it is essential. Listening has an active side which includes asking appropriate questions in order to clarify the information presented. It is only when you become a true learner that you can hear and interpret what the physician is saying. If you stubbornly hold to your own desires and agenda, you won't function as a learner-listener. You will filter what is said through your desires. You may hear only what you want to hear.

Before you enter the office, you need to ask yourself, "Who knows how to take care of my health best?" The question is not a blanket abdication of your personal responsibility to be a good steward. By no means! Moreover, hearing is not necessarily agreeing. Rather, asking the question helps prime the pump. It prepares you to be a learner. Only as you understand what the physician is saying and why he has drawn these conclusions will you be able to accurately interpret what he says.

What should a patient be listening for? Consider the following example from a typical day in my office that highlights the importance of listening. Ms. Patient comes complaining of pain and fatigue. She has assumed she has a body problem. Among other things, she says that problems in life are getting her down. She seems resentful and discouraged. After appropriate history taking and a physical examination, I make the diagnosis of soft tissue and muscular rheumatism which some equate with the diagnosis of Fibromyalgia (these conditions are common non-inflammatory and non-degenerative affecting the surrounding tissues of bone and joint).[5]

During our time together I ask her an array of questions. These include questions about her thinking regarding her body, her response to having a body that doesn't work like

---

5. See my website: jimhalla.com for free material addressing this topic.

she wants, and how problems of life (actually God's providence) may influence the way she feels (eventually and hopefully, we will address the connection between that which is outside of her and her feelings. In response, she may tell me that nothing is wrong with her thinking—"It's my body." She may even charge me with telling her that "it's all in my head." I ask her how she arrived at that conclusion. She said that other doctors had told her it was and, therefore, I was doing the same thing.

What are some potential problems in this scenario? From the physician's standpoint, I must determine if the problem is me and my delivery or is it her. I check myself to see if I have given an appropriate amount of information in a correct manner. Only then do I ask myself if Ms. Patient has come to the office as a learner. She may not have heard me because she was too busy focusing on something else. Or she may have heard me but misunderstood my questions or was uncomfortable with them.

Bottom line, Ms. Patient has not functioned as a listener and learner. She has based her response on conclusions drawn from previous encounters with other physicians. I need to be gentle and clear. Biblical listening on the part of the doctor and the patient always has the purpose of understanding in order to apply truth. Ms. Patient did not listen to learn. Christian or not, she needs to focus on understanding what I was saying. To function as a good steward (which only believers can do), she must listen to learn in order to be able to consider the validity and usefulness of what I was telling her. Ms. Patient had expectations and a plan on how to fulfill them. Good listening required her to set aside her plan at least long enough to understand what I said.

Consider another example. A patient told me this story: He went to a doctor with complaints of fatigue and pain. He had a history of several provable medical problems. The patient was upset because his doctor suggested he take an antidepressant. I asked him to help me understand his response. He told me that he wasn't depressed, that he had problems in his body, and that he had no reasons to be depressed. He had missed the point of going to his doctor as a learner.

My friend failed to have the doctor define for him his standard for the diagnosis of depression. My friend did not have to agree with the doctor's diagnosis or solution (in this case medication) but by not entering the doctor-physician relationship as a learner, he missed an opportunity to learn from the physician what led to the diagnosis. Was the diagnosis based on the description of my friend's feelings, his behavior, or abnormalities in the blood or other tests? My friend didn't like what he heard. He only wanted to feel better. By rejecting the diagnosis of depression, he failed to make a self-inventory and to consider how others perceived him. Consequently, he failed to consider the Bible as a resource for victory. Briefly, the Bible would point to feelings as a function of wanting and thinking. Unpacking the feelings would get to the thinking and wanting. With that approach by the physician or the patient or both, biblical truth would become practical, exciting, problem-solving, and God-honoring.[6]

---

6. For more on this subject, see my book, *Depression Through A Biblical Lens: A Whole Person Approach.*

The Bible has much to say about living a victorious life when our bodies are failing or when we feel like they are failing. Let's apply that truth to my friend. The doctor saw and heard something. But my friend did not utilize the situation to do a self-inventory and reevaluate himself according to biblical truth (James 1:22). If he had done so, he would have been in a position to rethink his perspective on and approach to living in God's world.

He would recall that from a biblical perspective, depression is an inner-man activity that is ultimately focused on self and control or a lack thereof. Feelings take center stage. Feelings are linked to thoughts and desires. The person, burdened down and drowning in a sea of feelings gives in to feelings and gives up on living and being personally responsible. These conclusions are based on his understanding about life (God's providence), himself, others, and God. Medical providers recognize that bad feelings produce bad behavior. They say the bad feelings are the basis for inactivity and physical complaints. The Bible, while no medical textbook, teaches that people are feeling-oriented, and function based on their feelings. Consequently, a person may cease to function responsibly and come to the doctor with a myriad of physical complaints. In cases such as my friend's, only the Truth and God's word will set him free (John 14:6; 17:17).

In effect, when faced with past or present unpleasantness of any kind, we are tempted to use bad feelings as a reason for not functioning and to explain our thinking, feeling, and acting. The Bible's view of feelings and thinking, however, stands in stark contrast to the definition of depression used by the medical field and the culture.

After processing the information, he heard from his doctor, my friend should make a problem list and ask himself where God is in his thinking. This vertical reference which is good theology forces him to practice good theology. Then he looks horizontally and asks himself how he might be self-focused. Having determined his thoughts, desires, and actions in response to each problem, he should compare his response to God's Word and find appropriate biblical principles that would help him respond to each problem by becoming more like Christ. In other words, he should use the Bible to interpret, but not necessarily agree with the doctor's assessment or the prescribed treatment. He is then ready to apply biblical principles to himself in his situation as he gets victory.

CHAPTER 12

The Patient as an Interpreter

A THIRD ASPECT OF FUNCTIONING as God's kind of patient is properly interpreting what has been said. Once you have listened to learn by gathering the facts, you are able to interpret (understand) what the physician has said. Facts are useful only if they are correctly interpreted and applied in solving problems. But note, consciously or otherwise, all facts are interpreted. Therefore, gathering facts is important, but something must be done with them. In one way or another, you will respond to them.

How you interpret what the physician says depends on your standard. Listening for and to godly wisdom is healthy (Proverbs 3:5-8; 13:14). On the other hand, the Bible calls interpreting facts apart from biblical principles foolishness and living according to one's own wisdom. Both of those responses hinder health (Proverbs 3:5-8; 10:21; 14:12). Therefore, you must decide between biblical wisdom and foolishness.

Jesus Christ is Truth (John 14:6) and God's Word is truth (John 17:17). That which is contrary to God's Word must be discarded. For example, take the following statements from various sources that you may hear as an explanation for a person's condition: "It is a physical problem, and therefore the Word of God doesn't apply." Or, "the problem is what is out there, and your response and feelings have nothing to do with your thoughts and motivations." Or, "getting relief is the essence of life, it is what you deserve, and any way you do is valid." Or "you are your circumstances and what you are and how you feel is a result of those circumstances."

These statements, too often accepted (or at least not countered) by believers, reflect the belief that personal responsibility to respond biblically to all of life (God's providence) including a hurting, failing body or any situation that is unpleasant, has been removed. Helping patients view and evaluate advice from a biblical perspective is one aspect of good stewardship. Such is one purpose of this book.

Consider the example of Ms. Hurt who is a seventy-five-year old, overweight widow with osteoarthritis (OA) of the knees. She visited the office because of knee pain and difficulty getting around. The physical examination showed changes typical for OA of the knee including quadriceps muscle weakness and atrophy. Radiographs of her knees confirmed an advanced stage of OA.

I presented the information that I thought she needed. She was listening intently and seemed to understand the diagnosis. Then I presented a treatment plan. The plan included the cornerstone of treatment for OA of the knees—quadricep strengthening exercises to be done at her home throughout the day and regular weight loss. The quadriceps muscles are the thigh muscles, and strong quads are essential to good knee function. Quad strengthening can reduce pain and improve function. But it requires a continuous effort on the part of the patient.

I discussed various other treatment options including total knee replacement. She stopped me short and firmly declared,

"No surgery." I asked her how she arrived at that decision. Among other things, she told me: "I am too old to have surgery."

Here was a lady who had listened to my diagnosis and the various treatment options presented to her. She had heard my interpretation of the facts (data that I had obtained from her history, physical examination, blood tests, and X-rays and my conclusion). I then set forth a plan by which we would implement a solution to her problem. She had interpreted the data, and she had arrived at a conclusion. However, that conclusion was drawn long before she came to the office. She said she based her "no surgery" decision on being too old and not wanting to be a burden to people. I could have stopped there but I continued to ask questions. Eventually she gave the bottom line answer which was twofold: fear and simply not wanting to have surgery. I asked her how old was too old. She didn't have an answer. Then, I asked her what would happen if she continued to decline as she had during the past year. She thought a moment and said she would call her family—the very people that she said she didn't want to burden.

She was oblivious to the fact that she was willing to put off surgery under the guise of not wanting to be a burden when, in fact, her failing body was becoming an increasing burden to herself and others. She was functioning as a poor steward of the body God had given her. "Not wanting to be a burden" as a major reason for not having knee surgery potentially led to her becoming a greater burden to herself and her family— and even the whole medical care system. The latter point is not to be ignored. It is easier and less expensive to prevent a fall and a subsequent hip fracture. Concern and love for her family demanded that she rethink her decision according to 2 Corinthians 5:9, 14-15 and Philippians 2:3-4.

Consider some of the implications as presented in Ms. Hurt's case. By helping Ms. Hurt apply the word of God I intended to give her hope and help. My goal was to lead Ms. Hurt into the joy and hope of godly stewardship of her body, her time, her situation, and her family. Certainly, there were things that she needed to do before considering surgery. She had weak quadriceps muscles, and she was overweight. But overall, she needed to think vertically which would help her to be a good steward rather than simply saying no to surgery. Being a godly steward would simplify her decision-making process as she cared for her failing body. When she did, life would be easier for her and those caring for her.

Even if Ms. Hurt was not a believer, challenging her decision by having her focus on others was useful. She was forced to reconsider her dependence on others. She wanted to stay at home as long as possible. By improving her ability to get around, she put herself in a better position to safely accomplish her goal of staying home. In addition, by approaching the situation from the standpoint of ministering biblical truth, I opened the door for further dialogue regarding biblical truth, both to her and her family.

In Ms. Hurt's case, I was not able to move any further than to remind her of Philippians 2:3-4 and its impact on receiving medical care not only for her benefit but for the benefit of others.

CHAPTER 13

The Patient as an Implementer

THE LAST ASPECT FOR US to consider in our study of becoming God's kind of patient is that of application and implementation. Not only should we listen to learn in order to understand, we must use the standard of God's Word to make proper conclusions. Then, and then only, will we be ready to apply what we have learned.

To be God's kind of patient requires a firm knowledge of what was said by the physician. This knowledge includes an understanding of your condition, the instructions of your doctor, and the practical steps you should take in order to live in a God-pleasing manner. Commitment to becoming a good steward is essential because living out your commitment requires patience and perseverance.

Let's consider several examples to help illustrate. Recall Ms. Hurt. I had given her an overall treatment plan. I explained to her what she needed in order for her to receive maximum benefit. I knew that if her goal was simply to gain relief, she would likely not initiate or fail to continue to be a faithful steward. If that happened, she would not improve and, in fact, she would deteriorate. But more importantly, she would not have pleased God.

You may ask if the physician has an obligation to help motivate patients in the right direction. Hopefully, you would
answer yes. The key is the definition of right. I spelled out what
I believe is God's definition of right in my books to physicians
(see footnote 2 in the Introduction). In Ms. Hurt's case, I began
to gently introduce biblical truth at a level and in a way that she
would be most receptive. I called on her to move away from a
self-centered approach to living by re-evaluating her decision
in the light of her family. That general approach holds for every
patient, and hopefully your physician will agree. Ask him!

Consider another example. As a rheumatologist, I hear a lot
about pain. Many patients are dissatisfied with their bodies
and their situation. The mantra I hear frequently is to function
"like I used to" without pain. Against sound principles of good
stewardship and against medical advice, some patients take to
the couch saying, "I have less pain when I am inactive." I term
these patients "couch potatoes." Others never stop. Like the
Duracell bunny, they go and go and go hoping not to think
about their problem, but which they are already doing. Their
approach to their physical problem is based on the premise
that they must accomplish so much in an allotted time. These
people I call "road runners."

Neither approach is based on a process that begins as a listening learner. Consequently, there is no proper interpretation
and application of what is said. Both approaches are based
on the patient's feelings and wants. One wants relief and is
willing to get it at any cost. His body will become more inef-
ficient over time and his function will deteriorate. The other
refuses to take stock of his condition and to develop a plan of
responsible living as a good steward.

Consider one last example. Some patients with chronic conditions such as rheumatoid arthritis or soft tissue rheumatism tell me that they grow weary. I want to know what they mean by growing weary and from what do they grow weary. The answers are varied but most say that having their body is a hassle to them. The body itself may or may not be deteriorating, but the person has grown increasingly uncomfortable. How do such persons display their weariness? Sometimes they stop taking medications and very often discontinue their exercise programs. When asked why, a frequent answer is that they have *forgotten* to continue these activities. In those situations, their commitment to godly stewardship and the application of biblical principles is found to be wanting, even non-existent— all to their detriment. Their life becomes more complicated, unpleasant, and more importantly, God is dishonored.

The Patient as a Theologian

HELPING YOU AND EVERY BELIEVER to seek medical care God's way is a primary goal of this book. A corollary goal is helping you minister to your doctor. Previously, we looked at the Bible's teaching on the subject of receiving medical care God's way. I gave examples of how a patient's theology influences his manner of receiving medical care.

Let me revisit the subject by clarifying a bit what I mean by the term "theology." Theology is sometimes defined as the study of God. But I am not speaking of theology in this manner. I am referring to applied knowledge or what some may call practical theology. Practical theology focuses on the application of the proper knowledge of God that enables us to live in God's world, His way, for His glory, and for our good. I am referring to the influence of the biblical knowledge upon our thinking, desires, and actions for all of life—including receiving medical care.

A patient's desire to honor God as a good steward is a theological activity that influences the type of patient he is. It is also a theological matter when a patient's desire for relief and avoiding bad health is placed above honoring God. In the first case, the patient is functioning as a good theologian, but in the second case he functions as a bad one. Certainly, then, the theology of a patient influences the kind of steward he will be.

When we consider *theology* as the influence of our relationship with Christ upon us in all areas of life, it becomes clear that theology focuses on relationships: God to man and person to person including patient to doctor and doctor to patient. Since believers, by definition, are in Christ by the gift of indwelling Holy Spirit, we are to grow in Christlikeness in every aspect of life. Relationships, both vertical (to God) and horizontal (toward man) matter. Relationships, good and bad ones, characterize living. Fortunately, and beautifully, the Bible focuses on relationships. Jesus makes this clear in Matthew 22:37-40:

> Jesus replied: "'Love the Lord your God with all your heart and with all your soul and with all your mind.' This is the first and greatest commandment. And the second is like it: 'Love your neighbor as yourself.' All the Law and the Prophets hang on these two commandments."

People respond to others and to God in various situations. A response to others is a response to God. Sometimes the response is attributed to the situation. Correct theology says that people and situations are not causative although they may be influential in a person's response. Responses can be either biblical or unbiblical. Developing relationships, good and bad ones, is a part of going to the doctor. Not only is a patient exposed to the doctor one-on-one, but he is exposed to the receptionist, nurse, and even other patients. How he conducts himself in those relationships have moral implications. How is that? We as believers are always in relationship to God and our neighbor. We need to consider the doctor, the office personnel, and other patients as our neighbors. Moreover, all relationships are moral and ethical because life is theological. Therefore, what we think, want, and do is to be in accordance with biblical truth. This is God's world and we are to honor Him in every aspect of life. Therefore, just as a physician's theology influences his care of his patients, so, too, does our theology influence how we function as patients.

CHAPTER 14
Theology Matters

I'VE SAID MUCH ABOUT THEOLOGY because theology matters. It matters because everyone is a theologian (everyone is a theologian because he has a relationship to God and has a belief about God), going to the physician is a theological activity, and we as believers are to honor God as patients and physicians. Moreover, everyone will function as a good or bad steward. These facts mean that our attitude toward God, our body, self, the physician, and office personnel influence how we function as a patient.

One way to determine if we are a good or bad theologian-steward is to discover how our response to the care we receive differs from that of the unbeliever. The goal that motivates us to go to the doctor, and the manner in which we respond to being a patient is a reflection of our relationship with Christ and its significance in our lives.

A. Listening and Theology

Think about listening. Every patient must retain a proper balance in the area of responsible listening. On one hand, some patients say something like this: "You are the doctor. Whatever you say goes." While a doctor may sometimes appreciate this response, the patient may in fact be abdicating his obligation as a responsible patient-steward. This *let go, let the doctor* attitude is like a *let go, let God* approach to growing as a Christian. In both instances, the person is functionally saying that he is not responsible to think and act in a God-honoring manner—the doctor or God must do it all. The prevalent idea of yielding and surrendering comes into play.

These terms too often indicate a passive approach which may be driven by fear, laziness, or an attempt to manipulate the physician to give some type of preferred treatment. In no way are we as believers relieved of our privilege and obligation to be a good steward. Regardless of the problem or the type of body that we have, God desires and expects us to practice good stewardship. It is best for every believer because it honors God.

On the other hand, patients may bring lists of medications and reasons for needing them. This approach can indicate *I am the doctor* attitude. Other patients may make demands on the doctor such as *just give me relief.*

None of these approaches acknowledges the following: the believer's obligation to be a good steward; the God Who providentially gave us the kind of body we have; God's help through physicians and medical technology. Being God's kind of patient requires that we properly balance our responsibility for being a good steward, with our attitude toward the physician who is to assist us in achieving that goal.

B. Maintaining the Proper Balance

Balancing the desire to please God as His kind of patient and choosing and depending on a physician begins with the person.

If that person is you, you must accept the responsibility and privilege for being God's kind of patient. In doing so, you will consider seeking out a physician who will direct you in the way of right stewardship. We have already discussed various aspects of stewardship.[7] For the believer, being a patient-steward means that we, out of gratitude for what God in Christ and the Holy Spirit have done for us, function as His kind of patient. Going to a physician simply because that physician is a good body mechanic may be poor stewardship.

Believers should find a physician who they believe will help them be good theologian-steward. The physician's own theology will influence his care of patients. We must be ever vigilant to distinguish truth from error by relying on God's word. This is especially true if the physician is an unbeliever. Sadly, that is often the case. Our churches must make it a priority to help develop physicians who will practice biblical-based medicine.

In our listening, we are to be quick to understand and to give the physician the benefit of the doubt as required by Matthew 5:9 and Romans 12:18. This will help to avoid communication problems. Too often patients blame their failure to understand on the physician. A good steward will work hard to understand the physician. Taking seriously the obligation and privilege of maintaining a right attitude toward the physician ultimately means "I have heard and reviewed your advice, asked appropriate questions, and I am in a position to evaluate it, and consider ways to apply it."

I am continually amazed at the number of patients who come to me for help but reject the treatment plan. Their

---

7. See Appendix A and B for further details.

rejection comes in varying forms. Sometimes patients are not interested in being good stewards. They consider the price of good stewardship too high. Such is the case of the patient with OA of the knees who refused to do quadriceps strengthening exercises, or the patient with soft tissue rheumatism who complains and "forgets" to do shoulder-shrug exercises and reports: "I am no better." Such is the case of a gout patient who continually "forgot" to take his medication and wonders why he continues to experience attacks of joint pain and swelling.

None of these patients are functioning as God-honoring stewards. They may have listened and even listened to learn, but either they have failed to correctly interpret what was said or they refuse, for whatever reason, to implement it.

C. Slander, Gossip, and Poor Communication

Let me mention a topic that is rarely discussed. Believers must not slander. If there is disagreement with the physician, they must attempt to reconcile with the doctor, not allowing the devil a foothold (Ephesians 4:26-27). To avoid misunderstanding, they must communicate possible disagreements clearly and gently. Disagreement between patients and physician or office personnel, handled in an unbiblical fashion, will lead to situations that breed trouble and dishonor God. Slander may even become fertile ground for legal action. This activity, especially between believers, is unbiblical. If need be, unresolved difficulties, for whatever reason, should be brought to the churches of believing physicians and patients for biblical resolution (see Matthew 18:15-18). The Bible insists that we must not solve problems in the same way as the culture

(Matthew 5:23-24; 18:15-18; 1 Corinthians 6:1ff). Desiring justice is not wrong. But using pagan methods to define justice and to attempt to get it, is wrong. Sadly, most churches refuse to help believers (including patients and doctors) to resolve matters between them.

CHAPTER 15
Wants, Desires, and Medications

AT THIS POINT, LET ME address a potential sticking point. I want to be understood clearly. I have been asked on several occasions if I am against going to the doctor for the use of medications. You may have concluded that I am suggesting it is wrong to want to feel better, to want to have better health, to want to have a better functioning body, or to want comfort. If that is your conclusion, it is wrong. Hopefully, based on the information presented so far, you have concluded that there is a right way and a wrong way to go the doctor. The all-important issue is for you to consider your motivation and the goals of going to the doctor, and the suggested method and means recommended in achieving those goals.

At issue is not the use of medications, per se, but the motivation of the patient and physician in using them. If medications are used simply to alleviate bad feelings, then the source of those feelings and the patient's response to them may never be addressed. Bad feelings often motivate a patient to visit the doctor. That in itself may be good stewardship. But from a biblical perspective receiving medical care requires that the believer consider the source of the bad feelings and enlist the doctor's help. Once the source of bad feelings is determined, then appropriate biblical solutions—including medicine—may be presented as part or as the whole of treatment.

Let's continue to think about the issue of good stewardship. We have been called to be good stewards of our bodies through the application of appropriate biblical principles. Therefore, consider James 5:13-16:

> Is any one of you in trouble? He should pray. Is anyone happy? Let him sing songs of praise. Is any one of you sick? He should call the elders of the church to pray over him and anoint him with oil in the name of the Lord. And the prayer offered in faith will make the sick person well; the Lord will raise him up. If he has sinned, he will be forgiven. Therefore confess your sins to each other so that you may be healed. The prayer of a righteous man is powerful and effective.

James concluded his letter by focusing on prayer. In verse 13, he asked if anyone was suffering hardship or trouble. If so, they were to pray. In verse 14, James broadened the concept of problems when he asked, "is any among you sick?" James taught that the individual who is sick has a responsibility. He is to call the church leaders who are encouraged to care for the sick by praying over them and by rubbing them with oil. James doesn't say what the content of the prayer should be. It may include a request for healing. But other Scripture passages must be consulted to address the content of any prayer including one addressing presumed physical problems.

The elders are to rub the sick person with oil (Mark 6:13; Luke 10:34). The use of oil was one of the best remedies for bodily ailments at that time. James is clearly advising the elders to minister medication as they address the whole person. God and science are not opposed to one another. God is the ultimate Scientist, Who established so-called natural and physical laws that He uses to govern our physical world and its activities. Faith and science are not antithetical, but they are intertwined because they both come from God. Therefore, improving the body and physical healing is not a matter of more faith as opposed to more medicine but a proper synchrony of the two. The choice is never between true science or saving faith. God never intended to separate the two. What God has joined together, man has no business separating. The problem is not science but the scientist and man's lack of understanding of God and His ways.

In verse 15, James addressed the results of the elders' prayer. Notice that the text referred to the prayer of the elders and not the prayer of the congregation or even the sick person. Prayer is a blessing and a privilege. It is communication with the Triune God through the Holy Spirit and by the intercession of Christ. Therefore, it is not to be misused. It is not an "open sesame" in getting God's attention to grant any wish. The truth is that nothing, including healing, is guaranteed. Rather, healing happens if God has decreed it. It is God Who heals not a person's faith or prayer. The prayer may be God's agent in the healing. Sometimes He uses medicine. At other times He says no.

James speaks of the distressed, sick Christian as being raised up by the Lord (verse 15). This raising up may include physical healing but not necessarily. There will be a deliverance from all physical problems for every believer in eternity, but the patient-steward may have to wait until then. Meanwhile, the believer is to function as God's kind of person. James' insight through the Holy Spirit should be a blessing and comfort for us as believers.

James added an important point. If the person has committed sin, he will be forgiven. The delivered and raised man will be a forgiven man as well. James taught that bodily problems may be caused by a person's sin. Psalms 32 and 38 are prime examples of bodily problems resulting from unconfessed sin. James is not advocating the philosophy that there is a sin behind every physical ailment or that confession of sin guarantees physical healing. But he calls the believer to confess any sin that may have occasioned the problem or any sinful response to the unpleasantness. James does not mean that every physical problem is due to a specific sin and confessing it is the key to unlocking physical healing. That would disgrace the cross and all believers who have never been healed. But sometimes sin does bring about sickness (see 1 Corinthians 11:28-32; Exodus 15:26; Deuteronomy 28:58-60; 2 Samuel 12:14-15).

Confession of sin doesn't necessarily remove the consequences of a previous or ongoing sinful activity upon the body (e.g.: liver failure due to the abuse of alcohol or emphysema because of smoking may not be removed simply because the believer repented and shows fruit of repentance such as cessation of drinking and smoking). Elders should inquire about possible sinful causes of the bodily problem. James' point is clear. He didn't consider the use of medicine and prayer alone to be effective in bringing about healing. James is calling for the patient to do a spiritual inventory (James 1:22). God is involved in healing. James knew sin can be at the root of some bodily problems, and often contributes to the problem.

In summary James is introducing the possibility of sin-engendered physical problems. James called for responsible action on the part of the elders and the sick person. The elders were to respond to the sick person's call. They were to pray over him and to apply proper medication. They were to inquire whether the sickness may have been the consequence of the person's sin. The Holy Spirit through James advocated prayer accompanied by medicine. James did not assume that the sickness was directly related to one's sin. But he did exhort the elders to examine whether this is so, thus ministering to both whole person—body and soul.

Sometimes medications are recommended to assist a person in getting relief and perhaps cure which may be evidence of good stewardship. However, and always, the use of medications must be directed by biblical principles. Some believe that changing chemicals in the brain by drugs (if that is in fact what happens!) changes man's moral compass. Man is a morally responsible being by virtue of God's original creation. In this sense, man as a morally responsible, ethical being is patterned after God. He is the image of God but not the Original! A believer's morality resides in his inner man (heart, mind) and is under the influence of the Holy Spirit and not medication.

The Bible is clear about the way to better health and a prosperous life. It is to fear God and to shun evil thus bringing prosperity to the body (Proverbs 3:5-8; 8:13; 14:16). Any approach to the care of people, especially those with physical problems that fails to apply this principle, is rebellion against God.

CHAPTER 16

The Patient's Expectations and Response When the Physician is an Unbeliever

THIS CHAPTER ADDRESSES THE ISSUE of a believing patient and an unbelieving physician. First consider the question: is it wrong to establish a relationship with a non-believing physician? In part, the answer rests on the person's reasons and motivation for going and the availability of various physicians (for example, insurance plans may restrict patient choice). Why would a patient seek out an unbeliever? Perhaps he hasn't considered the fact that going to the doctor is a theological activity. He functions as if any doctor will do as long as he is "good." A problem arises because the term good is never defined or is defined without the use of the Bible. Too often, good is defined as almost anything that brings relief. Being God's kind of patient is never considered.

If the reason for going is solely for the purpose of good stewardship, then certainly the patient's choice reflects a God-honoring motive. For instance, if the problem is thought to be related to the heart, and if surgery is required, good stewardship requires that we consider the physician's surgical skills. It is good stewardship to seek out a surgeon who is skillful in his field. We can best do that by finding out what physician has a creditable reputation among his peers and in the community.

On the other hand, it is not prudent to see a physician who is a believer but does not have a credible track record in his or her field. However, one must be very careful that gossip and hearsay aren't the basis for judging a physician to be less qualified. A believing physician who does sloppy work (please be careful with this declaration) is a poor witness for Christ and does not honor God in the use of his skills. Good stewardship requires you to verify as much as you can before you make a final decision.

A. Expectations

As we have learned, every patient (and physician) has expectations. It is helpful to remember that an unbelieving patient and physician think and act only as unbelievers. The Bible teaches that unbelievers are more concerned for and about themselves than others. They are rich in their own spirit and not in the in the Holy Spirit (Matthew 5:3). The Bible expresses the concept of *rich in one's own spirit* in a variety of ways including *wise in your own eyes, trusting in your own understanding,* and ultimately as pride (Proverbs 3:5-8; 26:5,12,16; 28:11). Therefore, as Proverbs teaches, they are not wise people; in fact, they are fools.

The unbeliever is motivated by whatever is most important to him and which offers to him success and comfort. For the unbelieving physician, it may even be helping people or developing a large practice. But ultimately, help that is not biblically-based is really no help at all. To think so, is to embrace Satan's lie.

B. Biblical perspective

When confronted with questions, an unbelieving physician may be upset, and even irritated, or he may be threatened when a patient voices a desire to seek a second opinion. Even if the desire for another opinion is based on the patient's faulty wisdom or wrong hopes and expectations, an unbelieving physician, and sadly often the believing physician, will not acknowledge the patient's responses (believer or not) as an opportunity for him, the physician, to grow and change.

Moreover, the physician is in no position to recognize that the patient's request, even demand, is an opportunity rather than a burden. The Bible teaches that hard situations are to be used to develop Christlikeness (Romans 8:28-29). The unbelieving doctor has no desire or ability for such personal growth. Therefore, he can't and won't help the patient in this area. Of course, the biblical purpose behind all learning is the application of biblical principles in order to bring about God's glory and the good of the believer. This truth is foreign to the unbeliever all the time and to the believing physician too often.

Believers should not expect the unbelieving cardiologist or oncologist to discuss or even mention your relationship to the One True Living God through Christ with you or your family as you face physical problems and perhaps impending death. The joy of resurrection life will be absent from any discussion. He can only offer that which science and the culture provide—medications and human wisdom.

If a physician does speak of spirituality, it may be in the form of god as you know him. His thinking goes like this: "We live in a generic world where all blues are gray, and all whites are gray. One color fits all. It is no different with respect to 'God.'" This thinking reflects his inner man. Don't listen to him! The idea is something like this: "Since spirituality is 'spirituality,' the inner 'you' seeks to gain some sense of direction for you. And since we are all going to the same place, any god will do." Thus, the unbelieving physician may mention or even refer you to some specialist, or higher power, or god as you know him, but he cannot point you to King Christ. Rather, the focus of non-biblical spirituality is relief, you, and your feelings.

In summary, the unbelieving physician will not be able to tell you how to get true victory in tough times. At best, his victory is hollow and even counterfeit. God's truth is not a resource for him. Therefore, when he is faced with a patient who is discontent in and with his situation, he has only the culture's counsel to offer.

C. The believer-patient's response

Sometimes unbelieving doctors conduct themselves in ways that bring a sense of joy and sense of comfort to the patient. He may act kindly and compassionately, may spend time with his patients, and may exhort his office staff to do the same. This may be a vivid contrast with the believing physician next door who is abrupt, even rude, condescending and who may be unskillful as well (although he shouldn't be!).

What should we think? Simply this way: God's common kindness is alive and well in His world (Matthew 5:43-48; Acts

14:17)! We can and should rejoice that it is God's world and that God wields His control so unbelievers don't always function as people opposed to God which is a manifestation of God's undeserved kindness!

How should we respond to an unbelieving doctor? We have covered the general themes of maintaining a proper balance between being a responsible patient and an I- know-best type of attitude. We should listen to learn and be willing to reflect on and properly use the information received from the doctor (for example, he may present corrects facts about how our body works).

In addition, Matthew 5:13-16 and the Great Commission (Matthew 28:18-20) apply. Going to an unbeliever for medical care necessitates a certain obligation on our part because we are to be salt and light in a dark world. As such, we are to illuminate—bring truth to people in a variety of situations. We have an obligation and privilege to provide light in the most appropriate way. Therefore, we are required to minister to the physician. How we do so must be tailored according to our relationship with the physician and the opportunities given by God. Prayer is a good start. We can pray for the physician and for wisdom and for the courage to be gently and lovely bold in seizing opportunities to use God's truth as we grow our relationship with the physician. Perhaps the best way to minister is to respond to hard times by showing the richness of God's truth as given in the Bible. Living out our confidence in the Lord rather than depending on the use of certain questionable medications and a desired outcome of cure or relief is the best means to demonstrate the significance and impact of our relationship with Christ.

CHAPTER 17

The Patient's Response and Expectations When the Physician is a Believer

ANOTHER ASPECT OF DEVELOPING A theology of being God's kind of patient centers on what a believer should expect and how he should respond to the physician who is a believer. Should we expect something different from the believing physician in contrast to the unbelieving physician? As is true for any relationship between believer and believer, the believing patient can hope and even expect but never demand the believing physician to bring God's truth in some form to bear on the problem. What that will look like will be different in each physician's office. However, both the believing patient and physician should be expected by the other to acknowledge that God's Word has much to say about all of life, including the receiving and the giving of medical care. Both should joyously act accordingly.

A. Using Hard Times

A core theological issue is the believer's use of hard times to grow and change into the likeness of Christ. Our condition or disease is not the only issue. In fact, it may not be the greatest issue. Our wants, fears, and expectations, all aspects of thinking and wanting, drive our response to physical problems. Our desire for relief may be uppermost and, therefore, not in keeping with good stewardship. Our response to something we don't want or not having something we want (for example, functioning like we previously did) may be the problem. A physical problem is one thing but our response to it is another. In fact, our response may worsen our physical problem.

Believing physicians are in a position to help us get victory in any number of ways. They have the opportunity and the resources (the indwelling Holy Spirit and the Word of God) to minister to us as a whole person. For the believing physician, the issue is helping the patient work out biblical solutions to problems (Philippians 1:6; 2:12-13; 2 Peter 1:5-10). In that way, we will grow and change as he helps us apply one of the lessons of the cross: using hard times to become more like Christ, which is the only true victory. If relief is the main goal, then both doctor and patient will have missed an opportunity to gain God's victory and experience the joy of pleasing God.

B. Spirituality and the Use of Medications

Given the current atmosphere, many physicians, and believers, have chosen to weave an eclectic mishmash into the practice of medicine as I have mentioned previously. In doing so, spirituality, has become just another treatment option. Even believing physicians, who correctly define spirituality as referring to the God of the Bible, may reduce the concept to one of many treatment approaches. Often, prayer becomes a means to call upon God to function as the patient's servant. As I have said previously, there is no power in prayer but rather in the living God to Whom we pray. The physician who prays but neglects the use of biblical stewardship principles differs little from his secular counterpart.

There are potentially many reasons for prescribing medications. The patient's physical condition may warrant proven therapeutic regimens (such as antibiotics for certain infections, diabetic medicines, and hypertensive medications). However, there are areas where medical science is speculative and offers only theory. In those cases, a physician may prescribe treatment that addresses only symptoms and feelings. Some physicians may say that they are relying on medical science, pragmatism, or patient demands to justify prescribing medication. In addition, the physician may use medications, because he is more enamored by what they are purported to do rather than by the power of biblical truth.

From the patient's perspective, churchgoing and prayer are touted as avenues to improve health rather than following biblical principles of good stewardship. Consequently, the worship of the True God is done to get rather than to honor Him.

Then, too, the well-meaning believer physician, concerned about his patient from a biblical perspective, may not know how to bring the whole counsel of God to bear. Therefore, God's truth doesn't enter the picture. I urge you not to settle for any of these counterfeit approaches to physical problems! Encourage your Christian physician to think and act as one.

C. <u>What Should the Believer Do?</u>

What we should expect is best not left to speculation. We should ask the physician his view of the Bible and how it applies to his practice of medicine. It would be helpful to develop a working knowledge of the physician's view of God and how his relationship with Jesus Christ influences his own life. You can begin by learning his view of James 5:13-18.

How to gain that information is another subject. Many physicians may not be amenable to this type of relationship. We must individualize our approach and meet him where he is. You may be thinking "how am I to do that?" My answer here is not an exhaustive one, but it is a start. Physicians, including myself, may send out an introductory letter to new patients telling about themselves and their practices. The letter may contain clues to help you decide what to expect. Another means is to look at the reading materials present in the waiting room. However, if the physician is in a large group, there may not be as much freedom in supplying proper reading material. Learning where a physician attends church may also be instructive. Often other patients may be a source of information but gathering information in this format must follow biblical principles.

The direct approach saves time and cuts to the heart of the matter. I think the place to start is their view of the Bible. Find out by asking their ideas about such passages as 2 Timothy 3:16-17 and 2 Peter 1:3-4. If they seem taken aback, it may be because they are not accustomed to having people ask these type of questions. It may be because of the way a patient inquires or the timeframe in which it is done. Or it may be that they don't have appropriate verses readily available for use in their daily lives and medical practices. In any event, I encourage you—don't give up! Most growing Christians, including physicians, should consider it a privilege to open God's Word and discuss it.

CHAPTER 18

Contemporary and Alternative Medicine

THE LAST TOPIC FOR US to consider in developing a proper theology of being God's kind of patient is the use of so-called alternative medicine which appears under the official title, Contemporary and Alternative Medicine (CAM). I refrained from commenting on the use or nonuse of cannabinoids. It is such an exploding and explosive field. However, the principles I set out in the chapter are pertinent to these substances as well.

A. Why Study this Subject?

As a physician, I see many patients taking various pills and engaging in activities hoping to prolong life, promote health, and feel good. As many as 40% of patients visiting the doctor are taking or have taken some type of CAM. Reasons given for this upsurge include the perceived failure and adverse effects of conventional medicine to yield cures, a desire to avoid "unnatural" products, the lack of time physicians spend with patients, and the fragmentation of medical care.

Users of CAM invest in what they believe will make them feel better. In most cases, this emphasis drives them to the doctor as well. Too often they have chosen to focus on improving or maintaining "better" health assuming they will get a better quality of life in lieu of becoming more like Christ. They may seek to be good stewards of their body, but they fail to understand the greater truth of the cross: to use failing bodies to honor God. Their focus ignores certain facts: resurrection life begins at salvation and points to and is the means of being in God's eternal presence; this fact should sustain the believer now. Heaven is an awesomely wonderful place and becoming more like Christ on this earth is a good God's means for moving believers home; our good God has providentially ordered His world to include hard times and failing bodies for our benefit; those hard times are to be used by us God's way for growing into Christlikeness. Therefore, it is reasonable, and even prudent, to study this subject.

B. Defining CAM

By definition, CAM are interventions that had not been taught widely in medical schools until recently nor was it generally available in US hospitals. The availability of CAM has radically increased. CAM is fast gaining acceptance and is even touted by some as a first-line treatment strategy. Several features regarding CAM should be noted.

First, CAM includes a vast number of treatment modalities such as acupuncture, aromatherapy, biofeedback, some chiropractic care, commercial diet programs (including high protein diets), energy healing (laying on of hands), folk remedy, herbal medicine, hypnosis, imagery, lifestyle diets (vegetarianism or macrobiotics), massage, megavitamin therapy, relaxation therapy, self-help groups, spirituality, yoga, and so on.

Second, since the rise of the youth counterculture in the 1970s, CAM use has been spiraling upward, indicating that CAM use is not a passing fancy.

Third, there is a lack of rigorous, scientific data confirming or refuting the claims espoused by manufacturers, promoters, and users of CAM.

Fourth, a cornerstone in CAM is life-energy therapies. These therapies are based on the notion that a flow of energy can be utilized for health and healing. Many of these life-energy teachings and philosophies are found in various religions: *chi* (*qi*) from Taoism and ancient Chinese medicine, *prana* from Hinduism, *Innate Intelligence* in chiropractic, animal *magnetism* and *invisible energy* from Mesmer (the founder of modern hypnotism), *vital energy* in homeopathy, and *subtle energy* from contemporary energy therapists such as Therapeutic Touch. They are founded on non-biblical thinking. The promoters of these therapies have made a radical departure from the mainstream of knowledge about the body, and they embrace the false religions of Eastern and New Age Mysticism.

Fifth, most CAM therapies are alleged, at least in part, to prevent future illness or to maintain health and vitality as part of lifestyle choices. Health promotion and disease prevention (not the glory of God) are the driving motives for the use of the product or technique.

Sixth, these therapies claim to change the body so that the person feels better. The person then conveys this subjectivity to others. Their philosophy is to emphasize a supposed inner force or inner intelligence. This force can be mobilized only from supposed right thinking, which comes from something the person does (such as mediation), eats (such as certain foods or herbs), or takes (such as some type of natural substance).

Seventh, there is a growing emphasis to integrate so called conventional medicine and CAM in hope of gaining the best of both worlds. Some medical schools have set up integrative programs in hopes of obtaining so called "evidence-based" medical facts to "prove" the effectiveness of CAM.

C. The Believer's Response

What should be said about the use of CAM especially among believers? Since all of life is theological, any philosophy of how to live is a theology. CAM is a theology and manufacturers, promoters, and users are theologians. What is the origin of their theology? Is the Bible their source? In answering those questions, consider the following.

First, when any treatment including CAM claims to offer long life and health, the believer must look hard to ascertain if there is a denial of sin and its effect on the body. Rather, God has exercised His prerogative in so judging and cursing sin and sinners so that the presence of all physical problems can be traced back to Adam's sin (Romans 5:12-14).

That is not to say that all physical problems are the direct result of a personal, specific sin, or that the person with cancer is being punished, or that he is a worse sinner compared to one without cancer. But it is to say that every person is joined to Adam representatively. Since Adam's sin in the Garden, everyone is a sinner and has been judged guilty and condemned by God. Therefore, by the sin of one man, Adam, misery and death flow to everyone (Genesis 5; Romans 5:12-14).

Second, when disease is present one reasonable goal of patient and physician is the correction of the disease state. This goal may be part of the practice of good stewardship by both patient and doctor. However, CAM seems to be an attempt to slow the effects of God's curse on sin based on the belief that CAM can do it.

Third, CAM has as its emphasis "the inner you" that can and needs to be mobilized for "your" health.

Fourth, CAM has as its focus the physical, the temporary, the material, and the personal in order to fulfill the hope, desire, and even demand of a lifetime of self-pleasure, health, and comfort.

Taken together, these principles show that in many instances CAM denies the biblical view of God, man, and sin.

Compare the teaching of CAM manufacturers, promoters, and users with that of the Bible. God saves His people by His re-creative activity (John 3:3-8)! God's sole purpose for saving people is to fulfill His original design for His people, which is for them to enjoy, glorify, and please Him, and to live in His presence forever (John 6:37-43; Ephesians 1:4). God's design of life after salvation is summarized as becoming more like Christ daily. We are to live out our present lives, using hard times as one of our tools to grow and change into Christlikeness. How does CAM help people grow and change spiritually? It doesn't. Since CAM has its origin and source in non-biblical thinking, it distorts God's truth, and moves people away from God's purpose.

D. Traditional Medicine

But before you think I am singling out CAM, look at the subject from another angle. How does CAM compare with conventional and orthodox medicine? From one viewpoint, CAM does not meet empiric, objective standards often required of medicine and devices, according to Food and Drug Administration (FDA) standards. While the FDA has its own inherent problems, it does serve the purpose of establishing some ground rules of objectivity. Subjectivity is the only standard for the success of CAM. Unfortunately, conventional medicine itself often follows this line of reasoning when it introduces and depends on subjectivity and behavioral changes as both diagnostic criteria and parameters for presumed successful treatment.

The published results of CAM are primarily composed of anecdotal evidence and testimonials which are based solely on a person's report of his feelings rather than the results of scientifically-designed studies with objective measures. Thus, CAM, and often conventional medicine, has a flexible and changing standard for judging the success or failure of a treatment. It is virtually impossible to say that the CAM did or did not do what the person said it did. The term placebo effect is well known and refers to a substance that is inactive and harmless. A patient reports "success" based on his thoughts and feelings after ingesting the substance even though the substance demonstrated no measurable on the body (see my blog series: Science and the Bible, four parts; website: jimhalla.com). There are no objective measures to judge results except perhaps a happy face. The placebo effect illustrates the relationship between thinking, feelings, and sense perception all of which are addressed in the Bible. But these facts don't seem to bother or concern the manufacturers, promoters, and users of CAM. Feelings reign.

The four considerations made previously regarding CAM, also apply to conventional medicine. Clearly, conventional medicine has its own problems. In certain conditions and instances conventional medicine seems to look more like CAM in terms of goals, methodology, and parameters of alleged success. Like CAM, if practiced using a secular mindset, conventional medicine denies the God of the universe, the curse of sin, and can be used by physician and patient alike to attempt to fulfill the inordinate desire and hope of health and comfort while on this earth.

Moreover, the current emphasis of conventional medicine on the immaterial aspect of man is in opposition to the clear teaching of Scripture. This is seen most clearly in those conditions in which no pathology is found. Subjectivity is the only criteria for diagnosis and success or failure of the treatment for CAM and many conditions treated by conventional medicine. For instances, in rheumatology, patients are often diagnosed with such conditions as Fibromyalgia and soft tissue rheumatism. A common diagnosis in a gastroenterology practice is Irritable Bowel Syndrome. Patients may be labeled as having a *psychosomatic* or functional disorder. What underlies all these conditions is the lack of abnormal pathology that can explain symptoms even when using a variety of techniques. And if an abnormality may be detected, it is not clear that the abnormality correlates with symptoms and signs. My plea is for everyone to apply biblical principles to every condition whether it is considered physical or not. When the believer does make that application, he will bring his thoughts, desires, and actions in line with biblical truth.

Conclusion

I HAVE PREVIOUSLY WRITTEN A book that addresses the practice of medicine from the doctor's side. The book in your hand is for you, the patient. Since all of life is theological and everyone is a theologian, practicing medicine and receiving medical care are not neutral activities. Attempting to exclude the God of the Bible and our relationship with Christ is impossible and it is functional atheism. The result is always bad for us initially and later because we dishonor God.

Having read this book, you are able to answer a number of questions that are pertinent to being God's kind of patient. First, is it ever wrong, even sinful, to not go to a physician and seek medical care? God's answer is yes—it very well may be wrong not to go to the doctor. The answer is based on the fact that our bodies are not ours—we do not own them. We will give an account to God for our care of them. Is it ever right to visit the doctor? Yes, when we go to the "right" doctor for the proper reasons.

Second, is our going to the doctor any different from our unbelieving friend next door who goes to the doctor? Does the fact that we are believers impact how we function as a patient? The answer to both questions is yes because we have been bought with a price and have a vital relationship with Christ through the indwelling Holy Spirit. We are set apart for service in God's kingdom. One way to serve Him is to function as God's kind of patient for His glory. A proof and testimony of His grace to us and our thankfulness is using what we don't like, often failing or seemingly failing bodies, to become more like Christ.

Third, specifically, how does our Christian faith influence the way we take care of our bodies? The scope of receiving care includes going to the doctor, our motivation and reasons for going, and our thoughts and actions, both at the doctor's office and after we leave. I have given many examples throughout the book that illustrate how to be God's kind of patient. Review those examples and add some of your own—both those that honor or dishonor God. Then aggressively pursue that which honors God.

Fourth, how does being a believer cause you to interact with the doctor? This last question forces us to look away from self. Perhaps you have never considered the fact and significance of whether your doctor is an unbeliever or believer. You should. We are to be salt and light wherever God places us. Ask yourself how you function in that area and reread the portion of the book that addresses this topic. If you have additional ideas, let others know and please—let me know.

May God bless as you apply the principles set forth in this book and thereby find satisfaction and contentment God's way.

APPENDIX A
All of Life is Theological

THE SCRIPTURAL BASIS FOR THIS statement is based on the following truths:

1. God is man's environment (Ecclesiastes 12:13-14; 1 Kings 8:27; Acts 7:48-49; 17:27-28; Psalms 24:-2; 139; 29:3-10; Isaiah 66:1; Jeremiah 23:23-24). This is an inescapable fact. God is not limited by space—He is present everywhere; therefore, there is no escaping God.

2. Man was created in relationship to God and a worshipper. Therefore, man had and has beliefs about God and himself. Every person is a theologian. In the Garden, Adam was a revelation receiver, interpreter, and implementer. God gave man information on how to best live in that relationship. Today it is no different because God provides His truth in the Bible.

3. Since God is in covenant with man, man is a covenant being, with covenant responsibilities, and he is entirely dependent on God. As a result, every person has a relationship with God and God with him, and he has beliefs about God which result in a lifestyle of thoughts, desire, and actions.

4. Man is an ethically responsible and moral being because man is God's image bearer, and God designed man in His likeness.

5. God's creation and His creatures are His and are therefore dependent upon and obligated to Him (Psalm 24:1-2; 29; 33:6-11; 50:7-11; 89:5-18; 93; 95:3-5; 104).

6. In the Garden before the Fall, Adam and Eve were in proper relationship to God and knew Him as Creator, Controller, Lawgiver, and Judge. (Genesis 2:15-17).

7. Unconverted man continues to know God as Creator, Controller, Lawgiver, and Judge, whereas converted man also knows God as Lawkeeper, Redeemer, and Father.

8. God saves in the context of relationships. His people were chosen in Christ before the foundation of the world (Ephesians 1:4). His people grow in that relationship as they become more like Christ—this growth is termed progressive sanctification (Romans 8:28-29; 2 Corinthians 3:18, 5:9, 14-15; Philippians 2:3-5).

It follows then, that every aspect of every person's life from beginning (birth) to end (man's destiny which is heaven or hell) and all in between (either growing in the likeness of Christ or in the likeness of Satan) is theological.

Characteristics of Biblical Stewardship

THE BELIEVER'S PRIMARY GOAL SHOULD be good steward-ship for the purpose of honoring God. Stewardship questions include: Will you go to the physician, and if you do, what is your goal? When there, what will be your relationship with the physician? How will you conduct yourself? Will you be a good listener? Will you be a good interpreter of the information and facts presented? Will you be a good implementer of that which you receive?

There are at least six characteristics of biblical stewardship.

1. God owns everything; yet, we possess what He has put in our care as a steward. We are to act as a good stew-ard under His Ownership. Stewardship begins with God. Therefore, biblical stewardship and taking care of our bodies is an ownership issue (see 1 Chronicles 29:10-20; Haggai 2:7-8; 1 Corinthians 6:19-20). Scripture emphasizes God's ultimate ownership as the Creator, Originator, and Controller of the universe. If God is not in charge, He isn't Owner. As Owner, He needs nothing. Yet He gives out of His abundance. God's ownership and His abundant giving are the twin pil-

lars for a proper understanding of stewardship. Unless there is right thinking about God, the Owner, and myself, the steward-entrustee will not function as God's kind of steward.

2. God entrusts to us everything we have, including our bodies. Therefore, stewardship is a responsibility issue (see 1 Corinthians 4:2-5; Psalm 139:13-16). How we possess anything is radically different from God's ownership. We possess things as a steward, not as an ultimate owner. Further, our possessing is temporary, and subordinate to God's ownership because we are not our own.

3. God owns everything we possess, but God gives and enables us to use it. This is a user issue (see Deuteronomy 8:16-18). How and what we think, desire, and do are theological and moral issues. Therefore, going to the doctor God's way is part of being a God-honoring steward.

4. God expects a return on what He has given. This is an expectation issue (see Matthew 25:14-30; Luke 19:11-27). In Biblical times, upon the master's return and perhaps after exchanging pleasantries, he would call his servant-stewards for an accounting. God is the Owner/Master Who will "settle up." God will judge us based on His view of our faithfulness as a steward. God takes stewardship seriously.

5. We must give an account of our care, and it may be today. This is an accounting issue (see Luke 12:16-21; Romans 14:10, 12; 2 Corinthians 5:10). Stewardship and accountability go hand in hand. Otherwise God would not be

serious about His ownership and giving. Either we are rich in returning to God what was rightfully His or we are sinfully holding on to what is God's for ourselves. In the latter case, we are stealing from God.

6. There are consequences, blessings and curses, for good or bad stewardship. Thus, stewardship is a result issue (see Matthew 25:24-27; Luke 19:24). God doesn't guarantee that our bodies will never hurt, fail, or become diseased on this earth. In fact, God has chosen not to reverse the effects of the fall and of sin on the body in this life (Romans 5:12-14). What He does guarantee is that stewardship His way is good for the believer. One way God judges a person's commitment to Him is through the grid of stewardship.

Believer, He bought you at the cross when His Son bled and died for you and every other believer. How can God expect anything less than a return on His investment? He can't! Therefore, honor God by being a good steward. It is best for you. Blessings as you do.

A Proper Understanding of the Terms: "Symptoms" and "Signs," "In the Body," and "With the Body"

THE TWO TRUTHS OF MAN'S duplex nature and the relationship of his inner and outer person should be placed along side of three important medical facts: symptoms and signs are not the same; symptoms indicate that something is wrong *in* the body, but not necessarily wrong with the body; signs often indicate that something is wrong *with* the body as well as *in* the body.

It is important for us and your physician to understand that symptoms and signs differ. Symptoms are subjective and depend on what a person tells the health care provider. Symptoms can't be verified or measured objectively. For instance, reporting a headache; "feeling bad," being depressed, down, or blue; hurting; being fatigued; being nervous; and feeling feverishness are symptoms. Their presence is based solely on what the person says. Feverishness is not the same thing as having a fever. A thermometer can indicate a fever, but it can't tell you if you feel feverish. Again, symptoms can't be measured objectively. There are no feverishness, pain, or fatigue "meters"—only what the person tells the doctor. That fact doesn't diminish the validity of the person's report.

The cause of a symptom and a sign is always related to the curse of sin. As mentioned above, they may be due to something wrong *with* the body or something wrong *in* the body. For instance, shortness of breath is a symptom. It may be related to heart and lung abnormalities. In that case, the symptoms are the result of both something wrong *in* the body and *with* the body. But the same symptom can result from a person's wrong thinking and wanting about himself, others, or the situation. In that case, there is something wrong *in* the body but not *with* the body.

Symptoms and signs develop because the human body is not flawless. The human body is sin-cursed and will never be symptom-free in this earthly life. Moreover, there will always be more complaints (symptoms) than causes discovered. This, in part, is related to limited technology and scientific knowledge.

On the other hand, actual tissue damage (disease) may be present producing abnormal cell and organ function that result in symptoms as well as signs (cancer in the lung which causes shortness of breath—a symptom, and fluid in the lung—a sign). Lastly, a person's evaluation of and response to circumstances in life may produce symptoms that are felt *in* his body. Signs such as a rapid heart rate and rapid breathing rate also may be the result of person's thinking and wanting. The bad feelings are symptoms and in the case above don't indicate that something is wrong *with* the body. They do indicate that something is wrong *in* the body.

A sign is a measurable abnormality noted on physical examination; it may or may not be reported by the person. For instance, the doctor may detect joint swelling or a joint contracture when he examines a patient. These are signs and indicate something is wrong *with* the body as well as *in* the body. In contrast, as noted above, a symptom is a description of how a person feels which can't be measured and which may or may not indicate that something is wrong with the body.

A symptom and a sign may not indicate pathology. As above, both may be caused by a body functioning normally (e.g.: a complaint of shortness of breath and a rapid heart rate or rapid breathing when the person is excited, fearful, going up and down stairs, poor conditioning, or exercising). In these cases, there is nothing wrong *with* the body in terms of disease. The rapid heart rate is felt *in* the body, but the body is not pathologically abnormal. On the other hand, a rapid heart rate may indicate that something is pathologically wrong *with* the body as when the patient has pneumonia, an overactive thyroid, or heart failure.

The distinction between something wrong *with* and *in* the body is very important for patients and physicians as well. Knowing the difference between the two terms helps any patient to be a good steward. Something wrong *with* the body may well describe a disease state that can be measured objectively (e.g.: rheumatoid arthritis [RA] or cancer). Either of these conditions produces both signs and symptoms which indicate that something is wrong *with* and *in* the body. The diagnosis of such diseases is not based on symptoms but upon finding pathology either on physical examination (signs), laboratory studies, or radiographic-imaging studies. For instance, a patient with RA may describe pain and fatigue which are symptoms but have signs of swelling and reduced joint motion on physical examination. The patient with lung cancer may describe shortness of breath and even chest pain. The diagnosis of lung cancer rests on finding of cancer cells in the lung tissue and not simply on the report of symptoms.

Conversely, as I have tried to explain, the phrase "something wrong *in* the body" refers to symptoms (such as chest tightness) or physiological changes (such as a rapid heart rate or rapid breathing rate). A rapid heart rate is a sign (it is measurable) that may be due to a variety of factors. If it is due to anemia (low red blood cell count) or hyperthyroidism (too much thyroid in the body), we would say that the findings are due to something wrong *with* the body. Bad feelings can result when there something wrong *with* and *in* the body.

However, as I have described previously, a rapid heart rate also may result from fear and worry in response to a certain situation. Or a person may "feel" as if his heart rate is rapid when in fact it is not. The doctor (and patient) should call the sensation a symptom. The resultant bad feelings can appear as if there is something wrong *with* the body, but in fact there is only something wrong *in* the body. Certainly, a person may aggravate something wrong *with* the body by wrong responses to problems in life including a failing body. By life I am referring to those situations and people that

God providentially brings into our lives. Good stewardship, therefore, requires attention to both the outer person and the inner person as we have discussed.

Most patients, and even physicians, too often, want to focus on symptom relief. If the problem is something wrong *with* the body, then treatment should be directed toward the physical abnormality rather than the bad feelings. Something wrong *in* the body requires a different approach, both by the physician and patient. When the problem is something *in* the body, most likely the body is working as it should. For instance, a person should feel bad when he has unconfessed sins or when he envisions problems bigger than God (Psalms 32, 38; Romans 8:35-39; James 5:13-18).

A. Further Clarifying Illustrations

Here are additional examples that help clarify the phrases "something wrong *with* the body" and "something wrong *in* the body." On physical examination, the doctor's fingers touch and sometimes poke various areas of the body depending on the patient's complaints. In response to the examination, a patient may report pain and even jump. Even this response by the patient must be evaluated under the theme of "something wrong *in* the body" or "something wrong" *with* the body. For instance, a person who reports pain all over his body and has complaints of pain upon the physician touching various parts of his body often will be diagnosed as having Fibromyalgia (this is the name given to patients who complained of pain and no abnormalities are found on physical, radiological, or laboratory exams). The areas that are reported to be painful by the patient are often termed trigger or tender points. The observation that these areas are painful rests solely on the doctor's interpretation of the patient's reported discomfort in response to the examiner's finger. In the case of the patient diagnosed with Fibromyalgia, something is wrong *in* the body, not *with* the body. However, the patient and physician must be aware that a response of pain by the patient may have other causes and could indicate that something is wrong *with* the body.

Conversely, consider the young child who comes to the physician complaining of abdominal pain. If the pain is localized in the right lower part of the child's abdomen especially when the physician releases gentle pressing, until proven otherwise, the child will be diagnosed as having appendicitis. In the child's case, there is something wrong *with* the body.

To further illustrate the connection between the inner and outer person, consider pain. Pain is physical; it is sensed or felt in the body at the pain receptor level that are located in the nerves of body's peripheral areas such as skin and muscle. Once activated, the pain signal travels along peripheral nerves to the spinal cord and up to the brain where the pain signal is interpreted. Therefore, it is inaccurate to speak of emotional pain, mental pain, or psychological pain. Emotions don't hurt. They are immaterial. There are bodily expressions that are called emotions (e.g: anger, fear). They emanate from a part of the brain, but they are whole-person responses that involve thoughts and desires. A person hurts but not emotions. I address this subject in section D.

Taken together these three terms are considered to refer to the non-material side of man. However, remember that pain is physical (material)—pain is felt in the body. There is little doubt that pain and its intensity are felt, and its presence and intensity are influenced by the person's thoughts, desires, and expectations which are both inner-and outer-person functions. Again, note the biblical truth of man's creation as a unit—the body, the outer person and the inner person, or the heart. Consider the following truths. Wants or desires which often become demands and thinking impact the body in terms of feelings and function; thoughts, desires/wants, actions, and feelings are linked. The Bible directs us to think God's thoughts and desire what God desires. Feelings and actions will follow. Feelings can't be the believer's guide whether patient or physician.

Moreover, the use of the terms emotional pain, mental pain, and psychological pain as a group refers to man as multi-compartmental (many parts) with presumed disorders of each part considered treatable by a variety of professionals. The terms are used to refer primarily to feelings (such as unpleasantness and discomfort) and hurts in a localized, specific portion of the person's make-up or total body complaints. We can say honestly that pain in not in a person's head as if it were only a bodily function. However, what is in a person's brain and more importantly in his inner person (heart) modifies the intensity of pain.

B. Feeling states often called (emotions) and the relationship between the inner man and outer man

I have used pain as a model for studying the connection between the inner and outer person. The unity of man of which we are speaking indicates that pain is a whole-person activity in the same way that anger, bitterness, sadness, and discouragement are whole-person activities. To speak of a person as "feeling angry" misses the point. A person feels angry because he is angry. Feelings are a person's perception of his whole person including his bodily state and the conditions around him.

Briefly consider the subject of emotions. The definition of emotion is fluid. No one field agrees on what an emotion is. Consider this description of emotions. Emotion, in everyday speech, is the conscious experience characterized by intense mental activity and a high degree of pleasure or displeasure. This description acknowledges thinking, wanting, and feelings. Scientific discourse has drifted to other meanings and there is no consensus on a definition. I favor calling an emotion a whole–person activity involving both the person's heart (inner person) as defined biblically and the brain which is part of the body. Emotions such as anger, fear, and anxiety are never neutral. They don't occur in the abstract. They occur in the context of a person's life, are felt in the body, and are linked to the person's thinking and wanting. So-called "emotional reactions" (emotions don't react people do!) are always associated with a person's view of his control and resources or the lack of both. They are expressed in response to how a person perceives what is going on around him and the God of those surroundings. Often this vertical reference is not considered or is denied by both patient and physician. The Bible teaches that so-called emotional reactions originate in the person's heart where he thinks and wants. In contrast, science teaches that these feeling states originate in the brain.

The foundation for the role of a person's attitude and feelings rests in the fact that God created man a unit. This means that stewardship must be directed at taking care of both your outer and inner person God's way. Stewardship is a whole-person activity, and a good steward will seek first to follow the Owner's principles given in the Bible. This is the most sensible and rational thing we as believers can do (Romans 12:1-2). In fact, to know God and apply His principles to all of life is the most beneficial activity we can do for our health (Proverbs 3:5-8; 4:23). Blessings as you do.

For more information about
Dr. Jim Halla
&

How to be a God-Pleasing Patient
please visit:

www.jimhalla.com
www.facebook.com/jimhalla
jimhalla@yahoo.com

For more information about
AMBASSADOR INTERNATIONAL
please visit:

www.ambassador-international.com
@AmbassadorIntl
www.facebook.com/AmbassadorIntl